Osteoporosis:
Prevention, Diagnosis, and Management

D0067951

Fourth Edition

Morris Notelovitz, MD, PhD

MB, BCh, FRCOG, FACOG
President Emeritus and Founder
The Women's Medical & Diagnostic Center
The Women's Research Center
Midlife Centers of America, Inc
The National Menopause Foundation, Inc
Gainesville, Florida

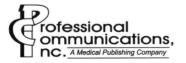
rofessional
ommunications,
nc. _A Medical Publishing Company_

Published by
Professional Communications, Inc.

Marketing Office:	*Editorial Office:*
400 Center Bay Drive	PO Box 10
West Islip, NY 11795	Caddo, OK 74729-0010
(t) 631/661-2852	(t) 580/367-9838
(f) 631/661-2167	(f) 580/367-9989

For orders only, please call
1-800-337-9838

or visit our website at
www.pcibooks.com

ISBN: 1-884735-84-3

Printed in the United States of America

DISCLAIMER

The opinions expressed in this publication reflect those of the author. However, the author makes no warranty regarding the contents of the publication. The protocols described herein are general and may not apply to a specific patient. Any product mentioned in this publication should be taken in accordance with the prescribing information provided by the manufacturer.

This text is printed on recycled paper.

DEDICATION

To my patients:
They have shown me that
osteoporosis can be conquered.

To Richard Mazess,
a pioneer in bone densitometry:
This technology showed me the way.

And to the many scientists who by their
dedicated research are unraveling the
mystery of bone physiology — the basis
of good medical practice.

ACKNOWLEDGMENT

I wish to acknowledge the contribution of my colleagues and friends involved in osteoporosis research. I have been able to successfully apply their discoveries and my observations to clinical practice.

My understanding of the pathogenesis and management of osteoporosis has been enhanced by my 19 years of experience with bone density testing and the expertise of excellent technical assistants—Rogene Tesar, Lynda McKenzie, Patricia Dixon, Sandy Durham, and Carol Thompson—whose help enabled me to formulate the clinical program outlined in this book.

As all authors know, assistants with good secretarial and typing skills are essential for manuscript preparation; I have two of the best: Cara Carroll and Lisa Gibson.

Finally, I would like to thank all of the staff at The Women's Medical & Diagnostic Center, the Women's Research Center, and my long-suffering family for tolerating my obsession: the prevention of osteoporosis and its relegation to history.

TABLE OF CONTENTS

TABLES

FIGURES

x

1 Introduction

Osteoporosis is a preventable condition. Although it is responsible for much morbidity and even death, primary osteoporosis is not a disease in the true sense of the word. For this reason, it is realistic to anticipate that in the foreseeable future, we will regard osteoporosis in a historical context, much as rickets and vitamin D deficiency are regarded today. Achievement of this goal will, however, depend on three factors:

- Educating the lay community about the importance of developing maximal bone mass before menopause
- Applying the principles of emerging facts regarding the biology of bone—in health and disease—to daily clinical practice
- Introducing easily accessible and reimbursable means of identifying women at risk for osteoporosis into the health care system.

Accomplishing these tasks will make effective primary *preventive care* possible.

Osteoporosis is a skeletal disease characterized by low bone mass and microarchitectural deterioration of bone tissue, leading to enhanced bone fragility and a consequent increase in fracture risk. Three main factors are responsible for the fragility of bone:

- Reduced bone mass
- Impaired repair of the microdamage caused by normal wear and tear of bone, with disruption in continuity of the plates in cancellous (trabecular) bone
- Falls.

Because disruption of the microanatomy of bone cannot be detected clinically (except with regional magnetic resonance imaging–enhanced technology), the diagnosis and management of osteoporosis rest primarily on the recognition of reduced bone mass. In this context, it is important to draw a clear distinction between the following:

- *Osteopenia*: Reduced bone mass due to inadequate osteoid synthesis; carries no implication about causality
- *Osteoporosis*: A skeletal disease characterized by low bone mass and microarchitectural deterioration of bone tissue, leading to enhanced bone fragility and a consequent increase in fracture risk.

Osteopenia is a risk factor; osteoporosis is the disorder. Osteoporosis has a much higher incidence in women than in men and occurs primarily after the menopause. It is also more common in white than in black women.

Bone mass is believed to account for 75% to 85% of bone strength. The primary goal is to recognize low bone mass (osteopenia) early, with the objective of achieving a high peak bone mass prior to the natural menopause and the subsequent age-related years of bone mineral loss. At present, the tendency is to look for and manage osteoporosis in postmenopausal and older women. However, the path to osteoporosis begins with the first menstrual period, a point of which all women — and their physicians — should be made aware (see Chapter 4, *Identifying Women at Risk for Osteoporosis*).

Since osteopenia can be regarded as a precondition to osteoporosis, the following steps can help prevent osteoporosis:

- Premenopause: Acquire maximum bone mass

- Perimenopause: Screen for osteopenia
- Postmenopause: Control bone mineral loss.

Osteoporosis has a formidable impact on the life and well-being of 44 million Americans. Ten million individuals are estimated to already have the condition and almost 34 million to have low bone mass (osteopenia). In addition, osteoporosis-related fractures added an estimated $17 billion to health care costs in the United States in 2001. The real cost for hip, spine, and other regional fractures is not known, but the cost is rising annually as the prevalence of osteoporosis continues to increase. Clinicians treat individuals; no price can be put on the physical and psychological long-term consequences of vertebral deformity and chronic back pain experienced by an otherwise healthy woman.

Because of advances in technology and in our understanding of the pathogenesis and treatment of osteoporosis, we now recognize that it is never:

- Too early to start prevention
- Too late to treat established osteopenia and osteoporosis.

Despite arguments to the contrary, selective screening of asymptomatic perimenopausal women to detect low bone mass is a cost-effective use of health care resources. By identifying women at high risk for osteoporosis at an early age, much can be done to enhance bone density through:

- Exercise
- Good nutrition
- A healthy lifestyle
- The selective use of hormone and other antiresorptive therapy
- Bone anabolic agents, such as androgens and parathyroid hormone (PTH).

Primary care physicians and gynecologists, in particular, play a pivotal role in preventing this condition. The treatment of patients with established or recurrent osteoporosis is best referred to internists specializing in bone metabolism. This manual will provide a practical and concise approach to prevention, diagnosis, and management of this disorder.

SUGGESTED READING

Cummings SR, Black DM, Rubin SM. Lifetime risks of hip, Colles', or vertebral fracture and coronary heart disease among white postmenopausal women. *Arch Intern Med*. 1989;149:2445-2448.

Cummings SR, Melton LJ. Epidemiology and outcomes of osteoporotic fractures. *Lancet*. 2002;359:1761-1767.

Dempster DW, Lindsay R. Pathogenesis of osteoporosis. *Lancet*. 1993;341:797-801.

Kanis JA. Osteoporosis and osteopenia. *J Bone Miner Res*. 1990;5:209-211.

Notelovitz M. Osteoporosis: screening, prevention and management. *Fertil Steril*. 1993;59:707-725.

Riggs BL, Melton LJ III. Involutional osteoporosis. *N Engl J Med*. 1986;314:1676-1686.

Tosteson AN, Rosenthal DI, Melton LJ III, Weinstein MC. Cost effectiveness for screening perimenopausal white women for osteoporosis: bone densitometry and hormone replacement therapy. *Ann Intern Med*. 1990;113:594-603.

2   The Physiology of Bone

Bone Compartments

Bone is living tissue. The skeleton serves three important functions:

- Scaffolding for the musculoskeletal system
- Protection of vital internal organs
- Metabolic reservoir serving:
  - Hematopoiesis
  - Calcium homeostasis.

The skeleton can be divided into two main compartments and types of bone (Figure 2.1):

- *Axial skeleton*: This refers to the spine and vertebrae. The bone in this region is primarily cancellous or trabecular (Figure 2.1-A).
- *Appendicular skeleton*: This refers to the long bones of the arms and legs. The bone in these areas is primarily compact or cortical.

At the end of the long bones, there is a variable regional combination of trabecular and cortical bone. For example, the ultradistal radius (1.5 cm proximal to the styloid process) consists of approximately 25% cortical bone and 75% trabecular bone (Figure 2.1-B); the midshaft of the radius (measured at two thirds from the olecranon to the styloid process) is 90% cortical bone. A similar variable composition is noted in:

- The femoral neck (Figure 2.1-C)
- The greater trochanter (Figure 2.1-D)
- The shaft of the femur (Figure 2.1-E).

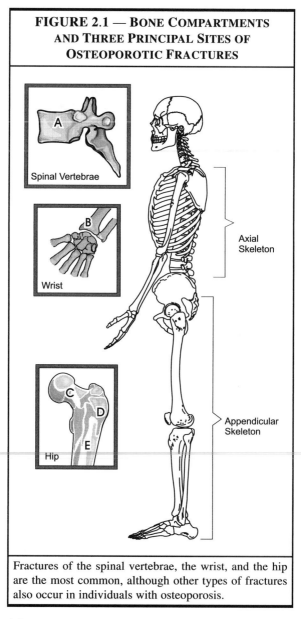

FIGURE 2.1 — BONE COMPARTMENTS AND THREE PRINCIPAL SITES OF OSTEOPOROTIC FRACTURES

A

Spinal Vertebrae

B

Wrist

C
D
E

Hip

Axial Skeleton

Appendicular Skeleton

Fractures of the spinal vertebrae, the wrist, and the hip are the most common, although other types of fractures also occur in individuals with osteoporosis.

The bone remodeling cycle is more active in trabecular bone; approximately 40% of trabecular bone is recycled annually vs 10% of cortical bone.

Because of the anatomic variability in these compartments, bone loss occurs more rapidly in trabecular bone (Figure 2.2), increasing its vulnerability to fracture. This explains why osteoporotic fractures tend to occur in:

- The vertebrae
- The femoral neck
- At the ends of the long bones.

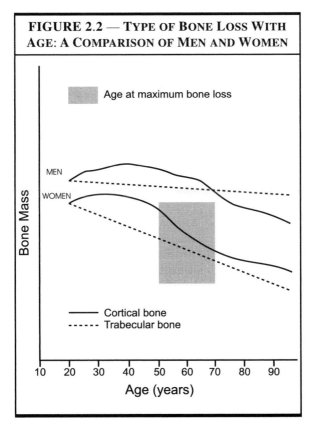

FIGURE 2.2 — TYPE OF BONE LOSS WITH AGE: A COMPARISON OF MEN AND WOMEN

■ Cortical Bone

Cortical bone has three surfaces (Figure 2.3). Each has different anatomic features but similar cell types and a similar bone remodeling cycle. The three surfaces are:

- *Endosteal envelope*: The surface facing the marrow cavity
- *Periosteal envelope*: The outer surface of the bone
- *Intracortical envelope*: Bony tissue between the endosteum and periosteum.

The activity of the bone remodeling cycle varies for each envelope depending on age and reproductive status, as follows:

- *Childhood*: New bone formation on the periosteum exceeds endosteal bone breakdown. A net increase in the outer diameter of bone results.
- *Adolescence*: Bone formation occurs on both the endosteal and periosteal surfaces with an increase in total bone mass.
- *Early adulthood*: Endosteal bone loss increases and begins to exceed periosteal bone apposition, indicating the beginning of age- or menopause-related decrease in bone mass, with a resulting narrowing of the intracortical envelope. The marrow cavity expands.

The haversian system (Figure 2.3) comprises concentric layers of lamellar bone arranged around a central canal containing blood vessels (also known as cortical osteons).

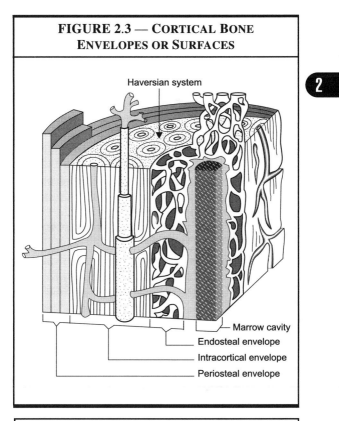

FIGURE 2.3 — CORTICAL BONE ENVELOPES OR SURFACES

Haversian system

Marrow cavity
Endosteal envelope
Intracortical envelope
Periosteal envelope

Clinical Message: The geometry of bone is now recognized to be a major factor in the etiology of hip fractures. Simple jumping exercises in young peripubertal girls significantly increase both the bone mineral content and the cortical width of the upper femur.

■ **Trabecular Bone**

Trabecular bone has a honeycomb-like arrangement of horizontal and vertebral plates that are interconnected. This ensures mechanical strength. Bone remodeling takes place on the inner and outer envelopes of each trabecular plate. Excessive bone remodeling results in thinning of plates, with eventual dissolution of tissue and loss of structural continuity. This occurs initially in the horizontal trabeculae and leads to a decrease in mechanical strength, with an increased liability to fracture due to physical stress (Figure 2.4).

> **Clinical Message**: Early recognition and interventions with appropriate therapy can maintain the integrity of the horizontal trabecular plates and — even in the presence of low bone mass — prevent fracture (Figure 2.4, *Osteopenia*).

Bone Remodeling

The renewal of bone determines bone strength. Old bone is "weak"; new bone is stronger. Bone remodeling refers to the removal of old bone and its replacement with new bone. Three classes of cells are involved:

- Osteoclasts
- Osteoblasts
- Osteocytes.

■ Osteoclasts

These cells are derived from the bone marrow mononuclear cells (preosteoclasts) that line the bone-forming surfaces. The characteristic feature is a ruffled border where active resorption takes place. The main function of osteoclasts is to dissolve bone mineral and digest bone matrix. The differentiation, recruitment, and inhibition of osteoclasts is controlled by numerous hormonal and growth factors (Figure 2.5). Osteoclasts have estrogen and androgen receptors; the primary effect of estrogen and other antiresorptive drugs is to inhibit osteoclast recruitment, function, and apoptosis (cell death). The introduction of the bisphosphonate class of drugs has led to a more detailed understand-

FIGURE 2.4 — CHANGES IN TRABECULAR BONE STRUCTURE AND BIOMECHANICAL COMPETENCE WITH AGE

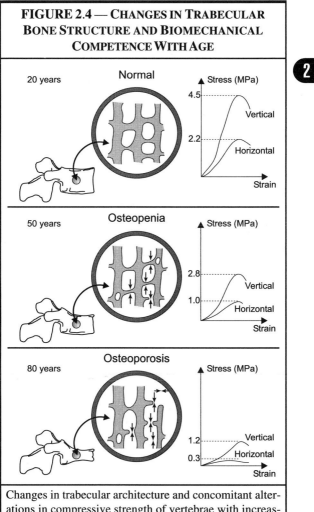

Changes in trabecular architecture and concomitant alterations in compressive strength of vertebrae with increasing age. Notice the initial preferential loss of horizontal trabeculae.

Modified and reproduced with permission from: Mosekilde L, et al. In: Takahashi HE, ed. *Bone Morphometry*. London, England: Nishimura/Smith Gordon, Niigata; 1990:367-370.

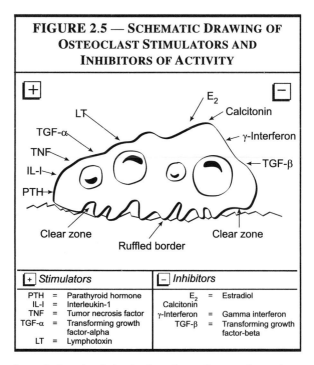

FIGURE 2.5 — SCHEMATIC DRAWING OF OSTEOCLAST STIMULATORS AND INHIBITORS OF ACTIVITY

+ Stimulators			− Inhibitors		
PTH	=	Parathyroid hormone	E_2	=	Estradiol
IL-I	=	Interleukin-1	Calcitonin		
TNF	=	Tumor necrosis factor	γ-Interferon	=	Gamma interferon
TGF-α	=	Transforming growth factor-alpha	TGF-β	=	Transforming growth factor-beta
LT	=	Lymphotoxin			

ing of the physiologic function of osteoclasts (see Chapter 12).

■ **Osteoblasts**

The main function of osteoblasts is to synthesize bone matrix (Figure 2.6). This is a collagen-rich (mainly type I collagen) ground substance essential for later mineralization by adherence of calcium hydroxyapatite and other crystals to individual collagen fibrils. Osteoblasts have estrogen and androgen receptors. Estrogen *in vitro* has the following functions:

- Increases the number of osteoblasts
- Increases osteoblast collagen production
- Increases nuclear progesterone receptors in osteoblasts

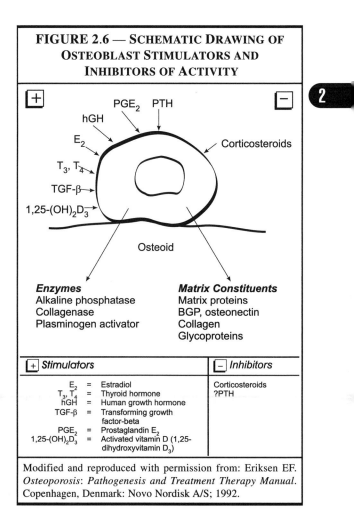

FIGURE 2.6 — SCHEMATIC DRAWING OF OSTEOBLAST STIMULATORS AND INHIBITORS OF ACTIVITY

+ Stimulators		− Inhibitors
E_2 = Estradiol		Corticosteroids
T_3, T_4 = Thyroid hormone		?PTH
hGH = Human growth hormone		
TGF-β = Transforming growth factor-beta		
PGE_2 = Prostaglandin E_2		
$1,25\text{-}(OH)_2D_3$ = Activated vitamin D (1,25-dihydroxyvitamin D_3)		

Modified and reproduced with permission from: Eriksen EF. *Osteoporosis: Pathogenesis and Treatment Therapy Manual.* Copenhagen, Denmark: Novo Nordisk A/S; 1992.

- Increases osteoblastic messenger RNA (mRNA) for transforming growth factor-β (TGF-β)
- Inhibits parathyroid hormone (PTH)–related increase in cyclic adenosine monophosphate (cAMP).

■ Osteocytes

Osteocytes are derived from the osteoblast lineage and produce nitric oxide (NO) and prostaglandins (PGs), both of which are responsible for osteogenesis by modifying the activity of osteoblasts and osteoclasts (Figure 2.7). Mechanical loading—exercise and gravity—regulates the quality of bone via the stimulation of osteocytes.

> **Clinical Message**: Exercise has been shown to enhance the bone-protective effect of estrogens and androgens. The same effect, based on physiologic principles, can be anticipated for other nonhormonal antiresorptives.

■ The Bone Remodeling Cycle

The bone remodeling cycle is a continuous process that ensures bone health and strength by coupling the removal of old bone (bone resorption) with synthesis of new bone matrix and later mineralization (bone formation). There are four steps in the bone remodeling cycle (Figure 2.8):

- *Activation*: Preosteoclasts are stimulated (by granulocyte-macrophage colony stimulated factor) and differentiated under the influence of other cytokines and growth factors to mature into active osteoclasts.
- *Resorption*: The newly formed osteoclasts secrete an acidlike substance from their ruffled border, dissolving and digesting the organic matrix and mineral of old bone.
- *Reversal*: Resorption ceases when the cavity reaches a predetermined depth. Monocyte-derived cells form a cement surface that prevents further bone erosion.
- *Formation*: Osteoblasts are attracted into the resorption cavity and, under the influence of various hormones and growth factors, mature to

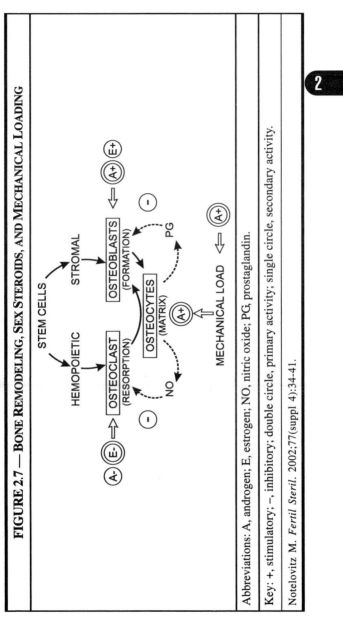

FIGURE 2.7 — BONE REMODELING, SEX STEROIDS, AND MECHANICAL LOADING

Abbreviations: A, androgen; E, estrogen; NO, nitric oxide; PG, prostaglandin.

Key: +, stimulatory; –, inhibitory; double circle, primary activity; single circle, secondary activity.

Notelovitz M. *Fertil Steril.* 2002;77(suppl 4):34-41.

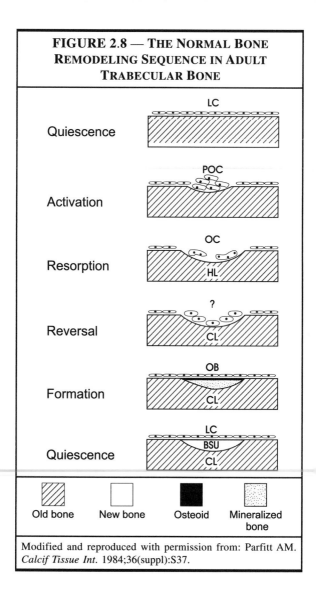

FIGURE 2.8 — THE NORMAL BONE REMODELING SEQUENCE IN ADULT TRABECULAR BONE

Quiescence — LC

Activation — POC

Resorption — OC / HL

Reversal — ? / CL

Formation — OB / CL

Quiescence — LC / BSU / CL

Old bone   New bone   Osteoid   Mineralized bone

Modified and reproduced with permission from: Parfitt AM. *Calcif Tissue Int.* 1984;36(suppl):S37.

refill the resorptive cavity with "new" bone. This takes place in two stages:

- The first stage involves the synthesis of bone matrix; 90% is made up of type I collagen. During the conversion from precollagen to collagen, extension peptides are removed. A serum assay for these peptides is available and can be used for monitoring bone formation. Two other noncollagenous proteins are formed that can also be used clinically as bone-forming markers: osteocalcin (bone GLA-protein [BGP]) and osteonectin. This glycoprotein "connects" the calcium hydroxyapatite crystals. BGP is made exclusively in bone, but osteonectin is found in other tissues. The collagen fibers are oriented in a triple-helix format and provide a scaffold for the later mineralization of the osteoid matrix. The type and maturity of the cross-links binding the collagen fibrils varies and is a significant predictor of the tensile (bendability) strength of bone.

Clinical Message: Newer assays are being developed that can measure modifications of the maturity (ratio between hydroxylysyl-pyridinoline and lysyl-pyridinoline [HP/LP]) and metabolism of the type 1 collagen molecule (isomerization/racemization ratio), and be used to predict the risk of fracture, independent of bone mineral density (BMD) and bone turnover rate. The variations in the degree of hydroxylation of the cross-links between individuals is probably genetically determined. Further, the type of cross-link may control the subsequent mineralization of bone.

- In the second stage, the newly formed osteoid is now mineralized with calcium hydroxy-

27

apatite crystals. The latter also contain trace amounts of magnesium, potassium, sodium, and carbonate. Two clinical points of note: (1) vitamin D_3 ($1,25\text{-}[OH]_2D_3$) is essential for this process; in its absence mineralization is defective, leading to osteomalacia; (2) the orientation and composition of the crystals and their resistance to osteoclast activity are altered by sodium fluoride. If sodium fluoride is used clinically, it is essential that adequate osteoid be stimulated, for example, by prior and/or concomitant estrogen and calcium therapy.

Bone Balance

(Figure. 2.9)

Bone mass is maintained when the resorption and formation phases are balanced (coupled). Negative bone balance (uncoupling) results from:
- *Overactive osteoclasts*: A resorptive cavity of excessive depth is created.
- *Impaired osteoblasts*: Inadequate osteoid is secreted to fill a normal resorptive cavity.

The accelerated bone loss in recently menopausal women is associated with enhanced osteoclast activity. The slower, age-dependent bone loss results from osteoblast underactivity. The net result is the same—bone loss.

Tests that identify the status of a woman's remodeling cycle are available, enabling clinicians to prescribe:
- Antiresorptive drugs, specifically in patients with high turnover bone loss

FIGURE 2.9 — POSSIBLE MECHANISMS OF FOCAL REMODELING IMBALANCE

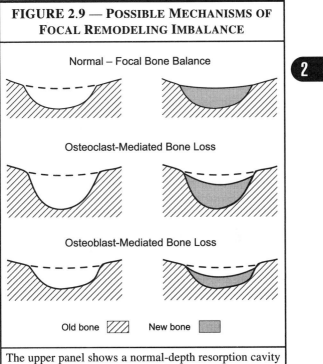

The upper panel shows a normal-depth resorption cavity on the left, completely refilled with new bone on the right. The middle panel shows a resorption cavity of excessive depth that is incompletely refilled by a normal amount of new bone. The bottom panel shows a resorption cavity of normal depth that is incompletely refilled by a subnormal amount of new bone. Note that the extent of net bone loss, indicated by the difference between the new and old locations of the bone surface, can be the same, despite the difference in cellular mechanism.

Modified and reproduced with permission from: Parfitt AM. *Med Times*. 1981;109:80.

- Bone remodeling stimulants in patients with osteopenia associated with low turnover bone loss.

At present, most drugs available for the treatment of osteopenia/osteoporosis are antiresorptive. Exceptions include sodium fluoride, androgens, and in the near future, parathyroid hormone (PTH).

Regulation of Bone Mass

■ Clinical Relevance of Peak Bone Mass

Peak bone mass, the maximal amount of bone mineral accrued during premenopausal adulthood (by age 35), is an important biologic milestone and serves two main clinical applications:

- The higher the peak bone mass, the lower the risk for subsequent osteoporosis. Thus women should be encouraged to achieve maximal premenopausal BMD.
- A comparison of the patient's current BMD with her peak bone mass helps in clinical management by allowing an estimate of the relative loss of BMD.

For example, informing a patient that she has lost 50% of her peak bone mass is an excellent incentive for that patient to accept treatment. An increase in BMD during treatment relative to the original BMD value at peak bone mass may encourage the patient to be compliant with prescribed medications and lifestyle.

■ Factors Influencing Peak Bone Mass

There are four major factors that determine peak bone mass (Figure 2.10):

- *Genetic makeup*
  - Ethnicity: White and Asian women are at greater risk

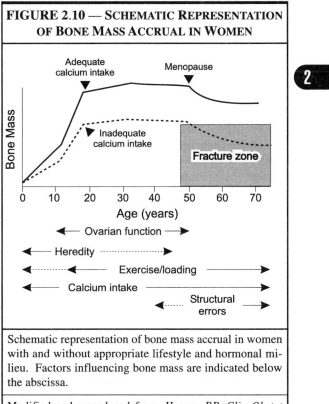

Schematic representation of bone mass accrual in women with and without appropriate lifestyle and hormonal milieu. Factors influencing bone mass are indicated below the abscissa.

Modified and reproduced from: Heaney RP. *Clin Obstet Gynecol.* 1987;30:833-846.

- Family history: BMD of young women significantly correlates with bone mass of their parents
- Monozygotic twins have BMDs that are more similar than those of dizygotic twins
- Polymorphisms of the vitamin D receptor, estrogen receptor, and collagen type $1\alpha1$ (COL1A1) genes have all been associated with reduced bone density. However, much of the variance in BMD is unexplained by these genetic variables.

> **Clinical Message**: Suspect low bone mass in daughters of women with osteoporosis. Concentrate on influencing their lifestyle.

- *Nutrition*: The protective effect of calcium is determined by the age at which adequate calcium intake occurs:
    - 75% of ingested calcium is absorbed in children; 30% to 50% in adults
    - Calcium supplementation in young adults increases BMD
    - Eating disorders (bulimia and anorexia nervosa) are associated with reduced bone density

> **Clinical Message**: Optimize good nutrition and eating habits in adolescent females.

- *Exercise*
    - Exercise stimulates the bone remodeling cycle. Bone mineral maintenance or hypertrophy of bone depends on the type and frequency of exercise and effects of gravity
    - Exercise during adolescence and adulthood increases BMD
    - Excessive exercise, which can diminish BMD, should be avoided, especially if this results in secondary amenorrhea
    - Exercise should be regular; osteogenic effects are lost rapidly if the intensity and frequency of the exercise decrease

> **Clinical Message**: Evaluate teenagers to ensure a regular and structured physical exercise program. Counsel them to avoid a sedentary lifestyle.

- *Hormonal status*: Reduced BMD is found in women with dysfunctional menstrual cycles:
  - Late menarche: The earlier the onset of menstruation, the greater the subsequent BMD; the later the menarche, the lower the bone mass.
  - Menstrual history: Women with irregular cycles have lower BMD. In one study, bone mass was reduced by 12% in women who missed <50% of their expected menses and 31% in women who missed >50% of their expected cycles compared with women with normal cycles.
  - Anovulation: Women with asymptomatic anovulation and no associated amenorrhea have lower bone mass compared with normal ovulating women. Bone loss with anovulation was estimated in one study to be 4.2% per year.

Clinical Message: Monitor women with late-onset menarche, irregular cycles, and anovulation/infertility. Emphasize nutrition and exercise, and, depending on the etiology, prescribe low-dose oral contraceptives.

■ Premenopausal and Postmenopausal Bone Loss

Bone loss is inevitable and is part of the normal aging process. Vertebral bone density may peak during the second decade. Bone loss is greater in trabecular than in cortical bone because it is metabolically more active and has a greater surface area.

Cortical bone loss occurs at the following rates:

- Age 40 to menopause: 0.3% to 0.5% per year
- One to 8 years postmenopausal: 2% to 3% per year.

Trabecular bone loss occurs at a linear rate of 1.2% per year from age 30.

Other Endocrine Factors Influencing Bone Formation

Alterations in the endogenous synthesis and secretion of various hormones and/or their exogenous clinical prescription can have a profound influence on bone physiology. Relevant endocrine factors include the following:

- PTH
- Vitamin D
- Calcitonin
- Thyroid
- Glucocorticoids
- Reproductive hormones.

■ Parathyroid Hormone

Parathyroid hormone is synthesized by the parathyroid gland. It has two biologically active terminals:

- The main activity is in the N-terminal end (PTH 1-34)
- The C-terminal end may have some renal activity.

Parathyroid hormone increases the recruitment and activity of osteoclasts and osteoblasts. If PTH secretion is excessive (eg, due to a parathyroid adenoma), the bone turnover will increase, but the bone mass will not be reduced since coupling remains intact.

However, where PTH secretion is enhanced in the presence of vitamin D deficiency and/or phosphate retention (secondary hyperparathyroidism), the bone remodeling cycle is accelerated with resulting bone loss.

Parathyroid hormone, if given intermittently, increases bone mass and has also been observed to induce reconnectivity of previously absorbed trabecular plates. It will soon be available as a treatment for osteoporosis.

2

■ Vitamin D

Activated vitamin D_3 (1,25-$[OH]_2D_3$) is formed by transformation from vitamin D_2 (25-$[OH]_2D$). The physiologic sites of action are:
- *Gut*: responsible for calcium absorption
- *Bone*:
  - Increases osteoclast recruitment
  - Stimulates osteoblast protein synthesis
  - Participates in mineralization of the matrix.

Lack of vitamin D results in impaired mineralization and osteomalacia. Excessive vitamin D can lead to bone loss.

■ Calcitonin

Calcitonin is produced by the C cells on the thyroid gland. Its main physiologic function is to inhibit osteoclasts. Pharmacologic use of calcitonin results in reduced bone turnover. However, it is only effective in patients with high-turnover bone remodeling. The bone-preserving effect plateaus after 2 years.

■ Thyroid

Thyroxine (T_4) and triiodothyronine (T_3) affect bone cells directly and indirectly via local growth factors, eg, insulin-like growth factor-1 (IGF-1). Hyperthyroidism results in:
- More resorptive sites
- Uncoupling, with resorption exceeding formation.

This leads to increased bone mineral loss and reduced bone mass.

Bone cells are very sensitive to exogenous thyroid, even in euthyroid doses. Patients on thyroid replacement should be monitored regularly with sensitive plasma thyroid-stimulating hormone (TSH) assays.

■ Glucocorticoids

Bone cells have glucocorticoid receptors. Excess corticosteroid activity results in:

- Inhibition of osteoblasts and, therefore, inhibition of matrix formation
- Decrease in calcium absorption with secondary hyperparathyroidism.

In patients on long-term corticosteroid treatment, their bone mass will be decreased. They should, therefore, have:

- Their bone mass monitored annually
- Urinary collagen cross-links assayed at regular intervals
- A compensatory increase in vitamin D and calcium prescribed.

Progestin inhibits steroid activity on bone and should also be considered in patients taking corticosteroids.

■ Reproductive Hormones
Estrogens

The two physiologically relevant estrogens are:

- Estradiol (E_2)
- Estrone (E_1).

In premenopausal women, E_2 is the predominant estrogen. In postmenopausal women, this is reversed, with E_1 becoming the predominant estrogen. An important source of E_1 is the peripheral conversion from androgen precursors, primarily androstenedione and testosterone. Most of this activity takes place in adipose tissue or in the relevant target tissue. This may be one reason why obese women are at a lower risk for osteoporosis.

Estrogen has a direct effect on all three major bone cells, primarily via binding to the estrogen receptor (ER), both α- and β-isoforms:

- *Osteoblasts*: *In vitro* effects include increase in osteoblast:
  - Numbers
  - Collagen synthesis
  - mRNA for TGF-β
  - Progesterone receptors
- *Osteoclasts*: Inhibition of bone resorption directly and (?) indirectly by a modulating effect of osteoblasts on osteoclasts.
- *Osteocytes*: Sensitization of the responsiveness of the osteocytes to mechanical loading.

The clinical effect of exogenous E_2 is dose-dependent. It may be that estrogen acts as an antiresorptive drug at traditionally used doses, with a bone-mass stimulating effect occurring at higher plasma E_2 levels. Indirect actions of estrogens include:

- Inhibition of PTH activity
- Stimulation of calcitonin secretion
- Increase in the gastrointestinal absorption of calcium (?) directly and (?) by renal activation of vitamin D_2 (25-$[OH]_2D$) to vitamin D_3 (1,25-$[OH]_2D_3$).

Progesterone

The role of progesterone in the physiology of bone formation is not clear. Progesterone receptors are present in osteoblasts following stimulation with estrogen. Progesterone (?) progestin blocks glucocorticoid activity in bone. *In vitro*, progesterone stimulates new bone formation.

Clinically, anovulatory (progesterone-deficient) menstrual cycles are associated with a 4.2% per annum bone mineral loss. Addition of progesterone to estrogen therapy may have a synergistic effect, increasing bone mass to a greater degree than with estrogen-only regimens. This is especially true for androgenic progestins.

Androgens

Men with hypogonadism develop osteoporosis; this can be prevented or treated with androgen therapy. Bone loss is due to uncoupling, with increased osteoclast activity similar to that seen in estrogen-deficient women. Bone turnover is decreased with androgen therapy.

Androgens play an important role in the physiology of postmenopausal women since they serve as the substrate for the peripheral source of estrogen. Oophorectomized women are affected more because of the loss of androgens produced by the stroma of the postmenopausal ovary.

Preliminary studies suggest that estrogen-androgen therapy may increase bone mass to a greater degree than estrogen-only therapy.

SUGGESTED READING

Arlot M, Edouard C, Meunier PJ, Neer RM, Reeve J. Impaired osteoblast function in osteoporosis: comparison between calcium balance and dynamic histomorphometry. *Br Med J*. 1984;289:517-520.

Banse X, Sims TJ, Bailey AJ. Mechanical properties of adult vertebral cancellous bone: correlation with collagen intermolecular cross-links. *J Bone Miner Res*. 2002;17:1621-1628.

Canalis E. The hormonal and local regulation of bone formation. *Endocr Rev*. 1983;4:62-77.

Dempster DW, Lindsay R. Pathogenesis of osteoporosis. *Lancet*. 1993;341:797-801.

Elders PJ, Lips P, Netelenbos JC, et al. Long-term effect of calcium supplementation on bone loss in perimenopausal women. *J Bone Miner Res*. 1994;9:963-970.

Eriksen EF. *Osteoporosis: Pathogenesis and Treatment Therapy Manual*. Copenhagen, Denmark: Novo Nordisk A/S; 1992.

Eriksen EF, Colvard DS, Berg NJ, et al. Evidence of estrogen receptors in normal human osteoblast-like cells. *Science*. 1988;241: 84-86.

Eriksen EF, Hodgson SF, Eastell R, Cedel SL, O'Fallon WM, Riggs BL. Cancellous bone remodeling in type I (postmenopausal) osteoporosis: quantitative assessment of rates of formation, resorption, and bone loss at tissue and cellular levels. *J Bone Miner Res*. 1990;5:311-319.

Eriksen EF, Mosekilde L, Melsen F. Trabecular bone resorption depth decreases with age: differences between normal males and females. *Bone*. 1985;6:141-146.

Garnero P, Cloos P, Sornay-Rendu E, Qvist P, Delmas PD. Type I collagen racemization and isomerization and the risk of fracture in postmenopausal women: the OFELY prospective study. *J Bone Miner Res*. 2002;17:826-833.

Heaney RP. The role of nutrition in prevention and management of osteoporosis. *Clin Obstet Gynecol*. 1987;30:833-846.

Kanders B, Dempster DW, Lindsey R. Interaction of calcium nutrition and physical activity on bone mass in young women. *J Bone Miner Res*. 1988;3:145-149.

McGuigan FE, Murray L, Gallagher A, et al. Genetic and environmental determinants of peak bone mass in young men and women. *J Bone Miner Res*. 2002;17:1273-1279.

Mosekilde L. Normal vertebral body size and compressive strength: relations to age and to vertebral and iliac trabecular bone compressive strength. *Bone*. 1986;7:207-212.

Mosekilde L. In: Takahashi HE, ed. *Bone Morphometry*. London, England: Nishimura/Smith Gordon, Niigata; 1990:367-370.

Nilas L, Christiansen C. The pathophysiology of peri- and post-menopausal bone loss. *Br J Obstet Gynaecol*. 1989;96:580-587.

Nottestad SY, Baumel JJ, Kimmel DB, Recker RR, Heaney RP. The proportion of trabecular bone in human vertebrae. *J Bone Miner Res*. 1987;2:221-229.

Oursler MJ, Pyfferoen J, Osdoby P, et al. Osteoclasts express mRNA for estrogen receptor. *J Bone Miner Res*. 1990;5(suppl 2):S203.

Parfitt AM. Bone remodeling and bone loss: understanding the pathophysiology of osteoporosis. *Clin Obstet Gynecol*. 1987;30: 789-811.

Parfitt AM. The cellular basis of bone remodeling: the quantum concept reexamined in light of recent advances in the cell biology of bone. *Calcif Tissue Int*. 1984;36(suppl):S37-S45.

Raisz LG, Kream BE. Regulation of bone formation (second of two parts). *N Engl J Med*. 1983;309:83-89.

Rodin A, Murby B, Smith MA, et al. Premenopausal bone loss in the lumbar spine and neck of femur: a study of 225 Caucasian women. *Bone*. 1990;11:1-5.

Schachter M, Shoham Z. Amenorrhea during the reproductive years — is it safe? *Fertil Steril*. 1994;62:1-16.

Seeman E, Hopper JL, Bach LA, et al. Reduced bone mass in daughters of women with osteoporosis. *N Engl J Med*. 1989;320: 554-558.

Seeman E, Tsalamandris C, Formica C, Hopper JL, McKay J. Reduced femoral neck bone density in the daughters of women with hip fractures: the role of low peak bone density in the pathogenesis of osteoporosis. *J Bone Miner Res*. 1994;9:739-743.

Welten DC, Kemper HC, Post GB, et al. Weight-bearing activity during youth is a more important factor for peak bone mass than calcium intake. *J Bone Miner Res*. 1994;9:1089-1096.

3

Clinical Types and Pathogenesis of Osteoporosis

Clinical Types

■ Primary or Idiopathic Osteoporosis

Women with osteoporosis in whom no definable medical condition is present are said to have primary osteoporosis. It is thought to result from an exaggeration of the uncoupling of the bone remodeling process discussed previously. Because the bone loss occurs postmenopausally, this type of osteoporosis is sometimes referred to as *involutional osteoporosis*.

Primary osteoporosis can be divided into:

- *Type I*, in which the bone loss occurs mainly in the trabecular compartment and is closely related to the postmenopausal loss of ovarian function
- *Type II*, in which bone loss involves cortical bone and is thought to be an exaggeration of the physiologic aging process.

This classification reflects the tendency for vertebral fractures to occur in women between 55 and 65 years of age, whereas femoral fractures occur in women over the age of 70. More than 40% of all women between the ages of 50 and 75 will experience an osteoporotic low-energy fracture. About 80% of osteoporotic fractures are involutional.

■ Secondary Osteoporosis

About 20% of low-impact osteoporotic fractures may be secondary to:

- *Medical conditions*, such as:
  - Chronic renal failure
  - Gastrectomy and intestinal bypass
  - Malabsorption syndrome
  - Multiple myeloma
  - Metastatic cancer
- *Endocrinopathies*, such as:
  - Hyperprolactinemia
  - Hyperparathyroidism
  - Hyperthyroidism
  - Adrenocortical overactivity
  - Diabetes
  - Hypogonadism
- *Connective tissue disorders*, such as:
  - Osteogenesis imperfecta
  - Ehlers-Danlos syndrome
  - Homocystinuria
  - Rheumatoid arthritis
- *Medications*, such as:
  - Anticonvulsants
  - Antacids (that contain aluminum)
  - Thyroid hormone therapy.

Pathogenesis

The changes that lead to weakening of bone and pathologic fracture vary according to the skeletal site and the underlying etiology. As far as the mechanism is concerned, there are three main factors:

- Irreversible damage to the microarchitecture of the bone
- Reduced bone mass
- An increased tendency to fall.

In older women, senile secondary hyperparathyroidism also plays a role.

■ Microarchitecture and Bone Repair
Trabecular Bone

Thinning and damage to trabecular bone can result from:

- Increased number of resorption sites, leading to transient and potentially reversible bone loss. The trabeculae are contiguous, hence mechanical strength is maintained. This condition is known as osteopenia.
- Increased activity of osteoclasts with pathologically deep resorptive cavities resulting in perforation of trabecular plates. The process is accelerated by resorption at opposite sites of the same trabecula with one lacuna penetrating into another. This degree of bone loss can only be diagnosed histologically. Microfractures will result in clinical fractures from minor trauma. At this stage, the condition is called osteoporosis. It was believed that new bone growth could not be stimulated to restore the continuity of perforated trabecular plates. This is now being challenged by new research involving intermittent parathyroid hormone (PTH) therapy.
- Decreased osteoblast function, with progressive thinning of trabeculae but few or no perforations (Figure 3.1). This will result in osteopenia rather than osteoporosis and may be reversible.
- Increased bone resorptive activity after menopause in some women, which makes them more susceptible to perforation of the trabeculae. Thinning of trabeculae is more common in men (Figure 3.1).

Cortical Bone

Cortical bone loss may be due to the following:

- Excessive endosteal activity resulting in thinning of the cortex and irreversible bone loss.

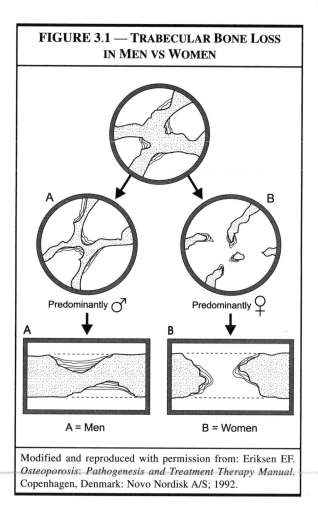

FIGURE 3.1 — TRABECULAR BONE LOSS IN MEN VS WOMEN

Predominantly ♂   Predominantly ♀

A = Men   B = Women

Modified and reproduced with permission from: Eriksen EF. *Osteoporosis: Pathogenesis and Treatment Therapy Manual.* Copenhagen, Denmark: Novo Nordisk A/S; 1992.

- Increased activity of the intracortical bone re-modeling units resulting in greater porosity of the cortex. The cortex remains the same, but is more fragile. This type of bone loss is potentially reversible.

■ Reduced Bone Mass
Osteopenia as a Precondition to Osteoporosis

Bone mass accounts for 75% to 85% of the variation in the ultimate strength of bone tissue. Studies confirm that reduced bone mass, irrespective of the site, is correlated with an increased risk for future fracture. Figure 3.2 places the role of bone mass measurement in perspective by conceptualizing the progressive thinning of the horizontal and vertical trabecular struts in individuals with osteopenia and its effect on bone strength. Mechanical strength is maintained with structural continuity of the plates (Figure 3.2-B). This stage of the condition is potentially reversible (Figure 3.2-C). Perforation and absorption of trabeculae result in subclinical microfractures and eventually overt vertebral fractures (osteoporosis). This stage is irreversible (Figure 3.2-D).

Microfractures are not clinically detectable (except by magnetic resonance imaging with microscopy-specific enhancement) and are best correlated with the degree of osteopenia. For example, treatment and correction of osteopenia (as measured by dual-energy x-ray absorptiometry [DEXA]) *are* associated with a lower risk for future fracture. Bone density is, at present, the best surrogate test. However:

- Densitometry may yield results that do not necessarily correlate with a corresponding increase in bone strength or meaningful increase in new bone formation.
- An increase in mineralization of the "stumps" of perforated trabeculae will result in increased bone mass measurement but not in a compensatory increase in the mechanical strength of the bone (Figure 3.2-E).
- Inhibition of accelerated resorption will result in the restoration of the original bone mass with an increase in bone density suggestive of new bone formation. This may merely reflect a res-

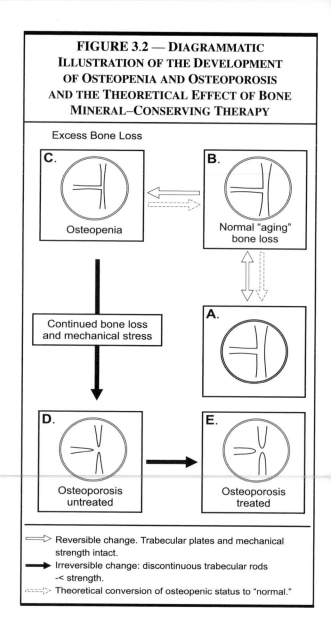

FIGURE 3.2 — DIAGRAMMATIC ILLUSTRATION OF THE DEVELOPMENT OF OSTEOPENIA AND OSTEOPOROSIS AND THE THEORETICAL EFFECT OF BONE MINERAL–CONSERVING THERAPY

Excess Bone Loss

C. Osteopenia

B. Normal "aging" bone loss

Continued bone loss and mechanical stress

A.

D. Osteoporosis untreated

E. Osteoporosis treated

⟹ Reversible change. Trabecular plates and mechanical strength intact.

➤ Irreversible change: discontinuous trabecular rods -< strength.

⤍ Theoretical conversion of osteopenic status to "normal."

toration of the bone mass by a "filling in" of the previous resorptive spaces.

- Changes may be due to bone age. Old bone has a higher mineral content. By slowing down the bone remodeling cycle (ie, with antiresorptive drugs), more old bone may accumulate with an increase in bone density. However, old bone has decreased resistive strength compared with new bone.
- Certain antiresorptive drugs (eg, raloxifene) may prevent future/further vertebral fractures by inhibiting resorption before perforation of the trabeculae and by maintaining this status quo without significantly increasing bone mineral density.

Bone mass loss (osteopenia) must, therefore, be seen as a risk factor for fracture but not diagnostic of the disease itself (osteoporosis). Nevertheless, depending on the site measured, there is a 1.5 to 2.5 increased fracture risk for every standard deviation below the norm for a given age group and bone site.

■ Falls: The Trauma of Osteoporosis

Most fractures are associated with mild-to-moderate trauma superimposed on low bone mass. This is true for both spine and hip fractures and is probably determined by the degree of underlying microarchitectural damage.

Persons who are especially vulnerable are those with a history of previous fracture. Women with two or more previous fractures have a 6.8 to 9.0 times greater risk of future fracture compared with women with no previous fractures.

The elderly are more liable to fall because of:

- *Reduced muscle mass and strength*, resulting in:
  - Slow gait with a tendency to fall backward instead of forward (Figure 3.3)

FIGURE 3.3 — SPEED OF WALKING AND THE DIRECTION OF FALLS

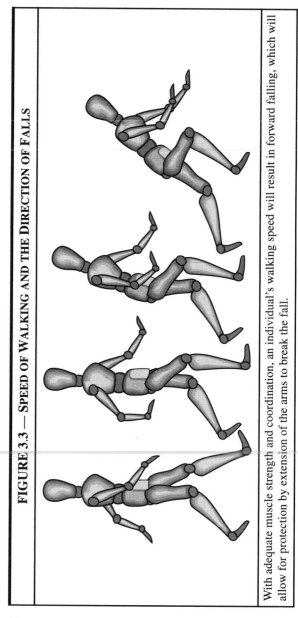

With adequate muscle strength and coordination, an individual's walking speed will result in forward falling, which will allow for protection by extension of the arms to break the fall.

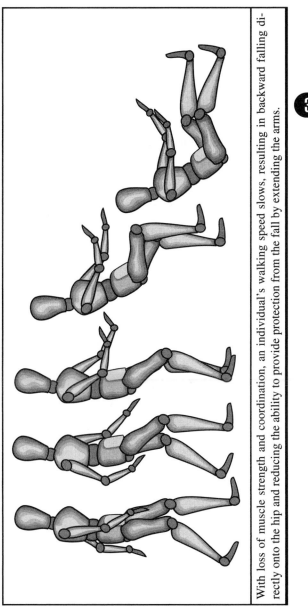

With loss of muscle strength and coordination, an individual's walking speed slows, resulting in backward falling directly onto the hip and reducing the ability to provide protection from the fall by extending the arms.

3

- Weak leg and arm muscle strength, which is responsible for the slow gait and the decreased ability to break the impact of the fall on the hip (Figure 3.4)
- *Reduced soft tissue*; soft tissue (fat) absorbs much of the energy generated by a fall and may be one of the reasons that obese women have fewer hip fractures. This is the basis for the success of hip protectors and the reduction of hip fractures
- *Central nervous system disorders* causing:
  - Slowing of reflexes

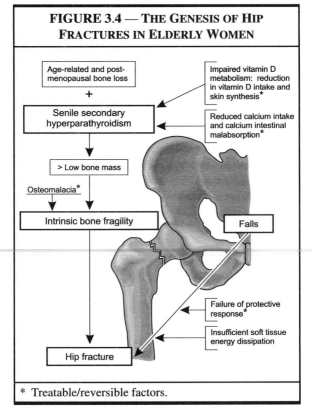

FIGURE 3.4 — THE GENESIS OF HIP FRACTURES IN ELDERLY WOMEN

Age-related and post-menopausal bone loss

+

Senile secondary hyperparathyroidism

Impaired vitamin D metabolism: reduction in vitamin D intake and skin synthesis*

Reduced calcium intake and calcium intestinal malabsorption*

> Low bone mass

Osteomalacia*

Intrinsic bone fragility

Falls

Failure of protective response*

Insufficient soft tissue energy dissipation

Hip fracture

* Treatable/reversible factors.

- Loss of equilibrium (vertigo and dizziness)
- Impaired proprioception
- Impaired vision and hearing
- Impaired coordination
- *Drug therapy*, such as:
  - Hypnotics and sedatives
  - Psychotropics
  - Alcohol.

Falls may be avoided when household hazards are eliminated. Steps that may be taken in the household to prevent falls include:
- Nonslip floor surfaces
- Good illumination
- Hand rails in the bathroom
- Beds and chairs easy to get into and out of
- No obstacles to trip over.

■ Senile Secondary Hyperparathyroidism

As women age, the serum PTH concentration increases. This secondary form of hyperparathyroidism is due to a combination of:
- Vitamin D deficiency due to:
  - Impaired metabolism, decrease in vitamin D intake
  - Reduced skin synthesis of vitamin D
- Low calcium intake due in part to an increase in lactose intolerance
- Reduced intestinal absorption of calcium.

This form of secondary hyperparathyroidism is preventable or reversible with vitamin D and calcium supplements. One way of identifying women at particular risk is to assay $25\text{-}(OH)_2D$ and if it is reduced, then measure serum PTH.

The contribution of senile secondary hyperparathyroidism to hip fracture is summarized in Figure 3.4.

SUGGESTED READING

Buchanan JR, Myers C, Lloyd T, Greer RB III. Early vertebral trabecular bone loss in normal premenopausal women. *J Bone Miner Res*. 1988;3:583-587.

Dempster DW, Lindsay R. Pathogenesis of osteoporosis. *Lancet*. 1993;341:797-801.

Eriksen EF. *Osteoporosis: Pathogenesis and Treatment Therapy Manual*. Copenhagen, Denmark: Novo Nordisk A/S; 1992.

Eriksen EF, Mosekilde L, Melsen F. Trabecular bone resorption depth decreases with age: differences between normal males and females. *Bone*. 1985;6:141-146.

Meunier PJ. Prevention of hip fractures. *Am J Med*. 1993;95(suppl 5A):75S-78S.

Notelovitz M. Osteoporosis: screening, prevention and management. *Fertil Steril*. 1993;59:707-725.

Nottestad SY, Baumel JJ, Kimmel DB, Recker RR, Heaney RP. The proportion of trabecular bone in human vertebrae. *J Bone Miner Res*. 1987;2:221-229.

Parfitt AM. Bone remodeling and bone loss: understanding the pathophysiology of osteoporosis. *Clin Obstet Gynecol*. 1987;30:789-811.

Riggs BL, Melton LJ III. Evidence for two distinct syndromes of involutional osteoporosis. *Am J Med*. 1983;75:899-901.

Riggs BL, Melton LJ III. Involutional osteoporosis. *N Engl J Med*. 1986;314:1676-1686.

Riggs BL, Wahner HW, Dunn WL, Mazess RB, Offord KP, Melton LJ III. Differential changes in bone mineral density of the appendicular and axial skeleton with aging: relationship to spinal osteoporosis. *J Clin Invest*. 1981;67:328-335.

Seeman E. Pathogenesis of bone fragility in women and men. *Lancet*. 2002;359:1841-1850.

Välimäki MJ, Tiihonen M, Laitinen K, et al. Bone mineral density measured by dual-energy x-ray absorptiometry and novel markers of bone formation and resorption in patients on antiepileptic drugs. *J Bone Miner Res.* 1994;9:631-637.

3

4   Identifying Women at Risk for Osteoporosis

Risk Factors

Identifying the patient at risk for osteoporosis is an important and often challenging responsibility (Table 4.1). Women traditionally considered most at risk are white or Asian, with a family history of osteoporosis and a petite, small frame. It was recently established that the bone density of young women is significantly related to the bone mass of their mother and father and that the peak bone density similar to that of their mother is achieved at 14 years of age. Monozygotic twins, with the same genetic modifiers of bone mass, are likely to have more similar bone densities than dizygotic twins. This is true at all skeletal mass sites measured, but the importance of the genetic effect diminishes with aging. The clinical message is to suspect low bone mass in the offspring of women with osteoporosis and influence their bone growth from an early age.

Lifestyle

Risk factors that are under patient control and may accelerate bone loss include:
- A diet deficient in calcium and containing excessive calcium-losing high-protein foods
- Inactivity
- Excessive use of alcohol
- Smoking
- Caffeine ingestion.

TABLE 4.1 — CHARACTERISTICS OF WOMEN AT RISK FOR OSTEOPOROSIS

Primary or Idiopathic	Secondary
Unavoidable: Race: White, Asian Family history Menopause Turner's syndrome Phenotype: small, fine bones Genetic polymorphism	**Medical conditions**: Chronic renal failure Gastrectomy and intestinal bypass Malabsorption syndromes Multiple myeloma
Accelerators: Nutritional factors: Calcium < Vitamin D >	**Endocrinopathies**: Hyperprolactinemia Hyperparathyroidism Adrenocortical overactivity Diabetes
Bone robbers: Caffeine > Protein > Fiber > Acidifying foods > Salt > Alcohol > Physical inactivity Smoking	**Medications**: Anticonvulsants Antacids (that contain aluminum) Thyroid extracts
Menstrual dysfunction: Late menarche Oligohypomenorrhea Exercise-induced amenorrhea Previous hysterectomy	
Eating disorders	
Scoliosis	

Gynecologic Factors

Women are especially at risk if they have had a premature or surgical menopause and have not received hormone therapy. Other gynecologic variables can also help to identify women with osteopenia.

■ Late Menarche

The onset of the menarche is an important biologic indicator of future bone mass: the earlier the onset of menstruation, the greater the individual's subsequent bone mass. With closure of the epiphysis, longitudinal bone growth ceases, but endosteal bone apposition continues for a variable period of time. Density increases markedly during puberty for both cortical and trabecular bone. Given the dynamic activity of the bone-remodeling cycle during puberty, this could be the optimal time to influence bone mass accrual with interventions such as exercise and nutrition.

■ Menstrual History

Cyclic disturbance of the menstrual cycle is an important marker of potential osteopenia. For example, in one study, women who missed <50% of their expected menses had a vertebral bone mass that was 88% of their eumenorrheic peers, and those who missed >50% of their menses had values that were 69% of the normal menstruating group. The plasma estradiol (E_2) values were lower and subnormal in both groups of oligomenorrheic women.

Women with asymptomatic ovulatory disturbance and no associated amenorrhea also have meaningful deficits in bone mass compared with normal ovulating control subjects. These changes are not associated with excessive physical activity. Bone loss in women with anovulatory menses is estimated to be 4.2% per year. The bone mineral loss is attributed to inadequate production of progesterone.

■ Exercise-Induced Menstrual Irregularity

During the past few years, a number of studies have documented the relationship between low bone mass and exercise-induced amenorrhea. This bone loss was thought to be reversible after activity was reduced and menses resumed. Unfortunately, the observed 6.3% improvement in one study slowed to 3% a year later and ceased during the next 2 years. A retrospective analysis revealed that a combination of extended periods of oligomenorrhea or amenorrhea and reduced body weight predicted 43% of the total variation in lumbar bone mass.

> **Clinical Message**: Closely monitor the thin oligomenorrheic or amenorrheic athlete.

■ **Hysterectomy**

Premenopausal women who have had a hysterectomy with retention of their ovaries have bone densities significantly lower than normal menstruating controls. It is not known whether this bone loss is due to aberrant functioning of the retained ovaries or to removal of the uterus per se.

■ **Extended Lactation**

Extended lactation is associated with bone loss. However, bone density may improve and return to baseline within a year after a woman gives birth. If breastfeeding continues longer than a year, the bone mineral density (BMD), although better, may still be significantly below the original value.

Eating Disorders

■ **Anorexia**

Patients with anorexia have significantly reduced bone mass compared with normal controls, sometimes even resulting in vertebral crush fracture. Neither estrogen nor vitamin D deficiency accounts for the bone loss in anorectic individuals, but physical exercise increases their bone mass to a level equivalent to sedentary normal control subjects. However, a follow-up study of some anorectic individuals found that 2 years of treatment with calcium, exercise, and estrogen resulted in most patients gaining weight but, unfortunately, no improvement in bone mass.

■ Bulimia

This eating disorder, which is characterized by binge eating and purging, is estimated to occur in approximately 1.3% to 4.3% of high school and university students. A negative correlation between bone density and purging with laxatives has been reported.

Other Endocrinopathies

Osteoporosis occurs in patients with hypoestrogenism due to gonadal dysgenesis (Turner's syndrome) and premature ovarian failure, irrespective of the cause. A less obvious cause of osteopenia is hyperprolactinemia. Significant bone loss has been reported in both cortical and trabecular bone, but not always in women with an associated estrogen deficiency. The pathogenesis of bone loss associated with hyperprolactinemia is unknown.

Scoliosis

Adolescent idiopathic scoliosis is a common problem with a prevalence of 1.8% if minor curvatures of 5° to 10° are included. Although the cause of scoliosis is not known, it is associated with a strong genetic tendency. Some studies have shown a relationship between hypoestrogenism and scoliosis. In a survey of 75 ballet dancers, the prevalence of scoliosis (24%) rose progressively with the delay in menarche. No fewer than 61% had associated fractures (mainly stress fractures), with the incidence increasing in those with secondary amenorrhea. Adult scoliotic women have a higher incidence of osteoporosis. Younger women with scoliosis should be regarded as being at greater potential risk for osteoporosis.

Risk Factors and Detection of Osteoporosis

Although the actual clinical significance of the factors discussed is open to question, a study that examined the risk factors for spinal osteoporosis in men showed that certain accelerators (eg, cigarette smoking and alcohol consumption) may increase the risk over and above that due to a primary causative factor.

In another study to determine the predictive significance of established risk factors when screening for osteopenia, the historical and bone mineral data of 859 women age 45 years and older who attended a screening program at the Center for Climacteric Studies (Gainesville, Florida) were analyzed. The following variables were considered:

- Height
- Weight
- Months of estrogen therapy
- Age at menopause
- Parity
- Months of oral contraceptive use
- Total and dietary vitamin D intake
- Total and dietary calcium intake
- Consumption of caffeine and alcoholic beverages
- Smoking
- Levels of alkaline phosphatase.

Bone mineral density and content were measured by single-photon absorptiometry. Statistically significant positive correlation coefficients (r) were obtained with height, weight, body mass index, age at menopause, and months of estrogen therapy. Significant negative correlations were found with elevated levels of alkaline phosphatase and increased cigarette smoking. Due to the large sample size, relatively modest r values yielded significant results. Accepted important contributors to normal osteogenesis (such as calcium, vitamin D, and exercise) did not contribute significantly to the variability in the bone density measurements. Neither did negative lifestyle factors, such as alcohol and caffeine consumption. The cross-sectional nature of this analysis and the use of a questionnaire to obtain historical data, with its obvious problems of recall, compromised the study. However, a more recent prospective study came to essentially the same conclusion: only 30% of the tested population could be correctly identified as having osteopenia without bone mass measurements.

Figure 4.1 is an example of a risk-factor questionnaire suitable for clinical practice. Utilizing a similar questionnaire, the National Osteoporosis Risk Assessment Study (NORA) evaluated 200,160 ambulatory postmenopausal women age 50 to 80 years from 4236 primary case practices. Using various peripheral BMD equipment (peripheral dual-energy x-ray absorptiometry [DEXA] of lower forearm or heel, single x-ray absorptiometry of the heel, or heel ultrasound), 39.6% of the study population had osteopenia (T-score of -1 to -2.49) and 7.2% had osteoporosis (T-score ≤ 2.5). Significant risk factors in the study included:

- Age
- Personal or family history of fracture
- Asian or Hispanic race
- Smoking
- Cortisone use.

The likelihood of osteoporosis was significantly reduced in:

- African American women

FIGURE 4.1 — OSTEOPENIA RISK-FACTOR SCREENING ANALYSIS

		Counselor's Review	
		Low Risk	At Risk

Name: _____

Date of Exam: _____

Age: _____ Sex: _____ Race: White/Asiatic/Black/Other

Height: _____ (inch) Weight: _____ (lb) BMI: _____ %IBW: _____

Reproductive Status:

Age at first period: _____ Date of LMP: _____

Regular periods prior to menopause: _____ ☐Yes ☐No

No. of pregnancies: _____ Live children: _____

Age of natural/surgical menopause: _____

Age ovaries removed: _____ Reason: _____

Years since menopause: _____

Fracture History:

Loss of height (more than 1 in) _____ ☐Yes ☐No ☐Don't know

Spontaneous fractures: _____ ☐Yes ☐No ☐Don't know

Bones fractured: _____

Family history of osteoporosis: _____ ☐Yes ☐No ☐Don't know

Medical History – Personal:

Osteoporosis _____ ☐Yes ☐No ☐Don't know

Rheumatoid arthritis _____ ☐Yes ☐No ☐Don't know

Overactive thyroid _____ ☐Yes ☐No ☐Don't know

Parathyroid disease _____ ☐Yes ☐No ☐Don't know

Gastrectomy _____

	Yes	No	Don't know
Chronic kidney disease _____	☐Yes	☐No	☐Don't know
Periodontal gum disease _____	☐Yes	☐No	☐Don't know
Chronic diarrhea _____	☐Yes	☐No	☐Don't know
Lactose intolerance _____	☐Yes	☐No	☐Don't know
Other _____	☐Yes	☐No	☐Don't know

Medication: 1 year or more

	Yes	No	Current	Past
Birth control pill: _____	☐	☐	☐	☐
Hormone therapy: _____	☐	☐	☐	☐
Diuretics: _____	☐	☐	☐	☐
Anticonvulsants: _____	☐	☐	☐	☐
Cortisone: _____	☐	☐	☐	☐
Antacids: _____	☐	☐	☐	☐
Thyroid: _____	☐	☐	☐	☐
Other: _____	☐	☐	☐	☐

Lifestyle: Daily

Exercise: _____	☐	☐	☐	☐
Consume dairy products: _____	☐	☐	☐	☐
Calcium supplements: _____	☐	☐	☐	☐
Smoke (more than 1 pack) _____	☐	☐	☐	☐
Caffeine (more than 5 cups) _____	☐	☐	☐	☐

(1 cup coffee = 4 cups tea, 6½ cups cola, 3 oz chocolate)

Alcohol (more than 2) _____   ☐ | ☐ | ☐ | ☐

(1 drink = 1 beer, 4 oz wine, 1 oz liquor)

4

63

- Women with a higher body mass index
- Women who take estrogen or a diuretic
- Those who exercise
- Those with little or no alcohol consumption.

Clinical Message: A number of other scoring systems, designed to select who not to test with BMD measurements rather than who to test, are listed in Table 4.2. The patient self-evaluation form (Figure 4.1) administered at the time of the patient's consultation (and reviewed by the physician) has been found to be simple to administer and interpret. In addition, it serves as a useful reinforcing educational tool for women. Risk-assessment programs and protocols can only provide guidance to both patients and physicians, but they can be optimally applied to helping the patient decide on the importance of having a bone density test.

SUGGESTED READING

Cadarette SM, Jaglal SB, Murray TM, et al. Evaluation of decision rules for referring women for bone densitometry by dual-energy x-ray absorptiometry. *JAMA.* 2001;286:57-63.

Davies MC, Hall ML, Jacobs HS. Bone mineral loss in young women with amenorrhea. *BMJ.* 1990;301:790-793.

Drinkwater BL, Bruemner B, Chesnut CH III. Menstrual history as a determinant of current bone density in young athletes. *JAMA.* 1990;263:545-548.

Gilsanz V, Gibbens DT, Roe TF, et al. Vertebral bone density in children: effect of puberty. *Radiology.* 1988;166:847-850.

Healey JH, Lane JM. Structural scoliosis in osteoporotic women. *Clin Orthop.* 1985;195:216-223.

Herzog W, Minne H, Deter C, et al. Outcome of bone mineral density in anorexia nervosa patients 11.7 years after first admission. *J Bone Miner Res.* 1993;8:597-605.

Howat PM, Varner LM, Hegsted M, Brewer MM, Mills GQ. The effect of bulimia upon diet, body fat, bone density, and blood components. *J Am Diet Assoc.* 1989;89:929-934.

Hreshchyshyn MM, Hopkins A, Zylstra S, Anbar M. Effects of natural menopause, hysterectomy, and oophorectomy on lumbar spine and femoral neck bone densities. *Obstet Gynecol.* 1988;72:631-638.

Johnston CC Jr, Slemenda CW. Risk assessment: theoretical considerations. *Am J Med.* 1993;95(suppl 5A):2S-5S.

Jonnavithula S, Warren MP, Fox RP, Lazaro MI. Bone density is compromised in amenorrheic women despite return of menses: a 2-year study. *Obstet Gynecol.* 1993;81:669-674.

Klibanski A, Neer RM, Beitins IZ, Ridgway EC, Zervas NT, McArthur JW. Decreased bone density in hyperprolactinemic women. *N Engl J Med.* 1980;303:1511-1514.

Lloyd T, Myers C, Buchanan JR, Demers LM. Collegiate women athletes with irregular menses during adolescence have decreased bone density. *Obstet Gynecol.* 1988;72:639-642.

Matkovic V, Fontana D, Tominac C, Goel P, Chesnut CH III. Factors that influence peak bone mass formation: a study of calcium balance and the inheritance of bone mass in adolescent females. *Am J Clin Nutr.* 1990;52:878-888.

NIH Consensus Development Panel on Osteoporosis Prevention, Diagnosis, and Therapy. Osteoporosis prevention, diagnosis, and therapy. *JAMA.* 2001;285:785-795.

Notelovitz M. The role of the gynecologist in osteoporosis prevention: a clinical approach. *Clin Obstet Gynecol.* 1987;30:871-882.

Pocock NA, Eisman JA, Hopper JL, Yeates MG, Sambrook PN, Eberl S. Genetic determinants of bone mass in adults. A twin study. *J Clin Invest.* 1987;80:706-710.

Pouillès JM, Trémollières F, Bonneu M, Ribot C. Influence of early age at menopause on vertebral bone mass. *J Bone Miner Res.* 1994;9:311-315.

Prior JC, Vigna YM, Schechter MT, Burgess AE. Spinal bone loss and ovulatory disturbances. *N Engl J Med.* 1990;323:1221-1227.

TABLE 4.2 — SELECTION CRITERIA SUGGESTED FROM THE NATIONAL OSTEOPOROSIS FOUNDATION PRACTICE GUIDELINES AND FOUR CLINICAL DECISION RULES FOR BONE MINERAL DENSITY TESTING AMONG POSTMENOPAUSAL WOMEN CONSIDERING TREATMENT*

Guideline/Rule	Selection Cut Point	Scoring System
National Osteoporosis Foundation (NOF)	Score ≥1	One point each for[†]: • Age ≥65 years • Weight <57.6 kg • Personal history of fracture: minimal trauma fracture >40 years • Family history of fracture[‡] • Current cigarette smoking
Simple Calculated Osteoporosis Risk Estimation (SCORE)	Score ≥6	Points are given for: • Race: 5 if not black • Rheumatoid arthritis: 4 if applicable • History of minimal trauma fracture after age 45 years: 4 for each fracture of the wrist[§], hip, or rib to a maximum of 12 • Age: 3 times first digit of age in years • Estrogen therapy: 1 if never used • Weight: -1 times weight in lb divided by 10 and truncated to integer

Osteoporosis Risk Assessment Instrument (ORAI)	Score ≥9	Points are given for: • Age: 15 if 75 years or older, 9 if 65-74 years, 5 if 55-64 years • Weight: 9 if <60 kg, 3 if 60.0-69.9 kg • Estrogen use: 2 if not currently taking estrogen
Age, Body Size, No Estrogen (ABONE)	Score ≥2	Points are given for: • Age: 1 if >65 years • Weight: 1 if <63.5 kg • Estrogen use: 1 if never used oral contraceptives or no estrogen therapy for at least 6 months
Body weight criterion	—	Weight <70 kg

* ORAI is also applicable for use in premenopausal women aged 45 years or older.

† For the purpose of the area under the receiver operating characteristic (AUROC) curve analysis, each factor was given 1 point. All those with at least 1 "NOF point" were identified for testing.

‡ NOF guidelines stipulate maternal/paternal history of hip, wrist, or spine fracture when the parent was 50 years of age or older. These specific data were not collected in CaMos.

§ Forearm and wrist were included as a history of wrist fracture.

Cadarette SM, et al. *JAMA.* 2001;286:57-63.

Rigotti NA, Neer RM, Skates SJ, Herzog DB, Nussbaum SR. The clinical course of osteoporosis in anorexia nervosa. A longitudinal study of cortical bone mass. *JAMA*. 1991;265:1133-1138.

Rigotti NA, Nussbaum SR, Herzog DB, Neer RM. Osteoporosis in women with anorexia nervosa. *N Engl J Med*. 1984;311:1601-1606.

Rosenthal DI, Mayo-Smith W, Hayes CW, et al. Age and bone mass in premenopausal women. *J Bone Miner Res*. 1989;4:533-538.

Screening for adolescent idiopathic scoliosis. Policy statement. US Preventive Services Task Force. *JAMA*. 1993;269:2664-2666.

Seeman E, Melton LJ III, O'Fallon WM, Riggs BL. Risk factors for spinal osteoporosis in men. *Am J Med*. 1983;75:977-983.

Siris ES, Miller PD, Barrett-Connor E, et al. Identification and fracture outcomes of undiagnosed low bone mineral density in postmenopausal women: results from the National Osteoporosis Risk Assessment. *JAMA*. 2001;286:2815-2822.

Slemenda CW, Christian JC, Williams CJ, Norton JA, Johnston CC Jr. Genetic determinants of bone mass in adult women: a reevaluation of the twin model and the potential importance of gene interaction on heritability estimates. *J Bone Miner Res*. 1991;6:561-567.

Slemenda CW, Hui SL, Longcope C, Wellman H, Johnston CC Jr. Predictors of bone mass in perimenopausal women. A prospective study of clinical data using photon absorptiometry. *Ann Intern Med*. 1990;112:96-101.

Soroko SB, Barrett-Connor E, Edelstein SL, Kritz-Silverstein D. Family history of osteoporosis and bone mineral density at the axial skeleton: the Rancho Bernardo Study. *J Bone Miner Res*. 1994; 9:761-769.

Sowers M, Corton G, Shapiro B, et al. Changes in bone density with lactation. *JAMA*. 1993;269:3130-3135.

Warren MP, Brooks-Gunn J, Hamilton LH, Warren LF, Hamilton WG. Scoliosis and fractures in young ballet dancers. Relation to delayed menarche and secondary amenorrhea. *N Engl J Med*. 1986;314:1348-1353.

5   Measuring Bone Mass

Bone Mass and Fracture Risk

After a decade of disagreement among experts, a consensus has been reached about the role of bone densitometry in the management of osteoporosis, summarized in the consensus statement issued by the National Osteoporosis Foundation (Table 5.1). Bone mass accounts for 75% to 85% of the variation in the ultimate strength of bone tissue. Compared with serum cholesterol measurements, bone density is a better predictor for osteoporosis than hypercholesterolemia is for cardiovascular disease. Also, bone density has a better degree of precision; 1% to 4% compared with approximately 10% degree of precision for cholesterol.

The contribution of bone mass measurement to estimating the remaining lifetime probability of fracture is summarized in Figure 5.1.

The earlier controversy stemmed from two main problems. First was the assumption that reduced bone density (osteopenia) was a reflection of existing fractures rather than a risk factor for osteoporosis. Studies now confirm that reduced bone mass, irrespective of the site of measurement, is correlated with an increased risk for future fracture. In one study, for each 0.1-g/cm decrease in the bone mass from baseline, the fracture risk increased 1.5 to 2 times. This is remarkably consistent with the conclusion of another study that the risk of hip fracture increased 1.6-fold for each standard deviation (SD) below mean bone mineral density (BMD) in the ultradistal radius. Although peripheral densitometry is predictive of hip and spine fractures and may be suitable for screening, hip and vertebral fractures are more strongly associated with bone

TABLE 5.1 — INDICATIONS FOR BONE MASS MEASUREMENT

- In estrogen-deficient women, to diagnose significantly low bone mass to make decisions about hormone replacement therapy

- In patients with vertebral abnormalities or roentgenographic osteopenia, to diagnose spinal osteoporosis to make decisions about further diagnostic evaluation and therapy

- In patients receiving long-term glucocorticoid therapy, to diagnose low bone mass to adjust therapy

- In patients with primary asymptomatic hyperparathyroidism, to diagnose low bone mass to identify those at risk of severe skeletal disease who may be candidates for surgical intervention

Potenial Indications

- Universal screening for osteoporosis prophylaxis

- Monitoring bone mass to assess efficacy of therapy

- Identifying women who are "fast bone losers" for more aggressive therapy

Clinical indications for bone mass measurements. Scientific Advisory Board of the National Osteoporosis Foundation. *J Bone Miner Res.* 1989;4(suppl 2):1-28.

density of the directly measured proximal femur and vertebrae, respectively.

The second problem was the inability to establish normative bone density values for healthy older women, and hence to quantify the definition of osteopenia. Two ways of quantifying bone density have recently been proposed. An individual's bone density can be compared with the mean and standard deviation (SD) of bone density for same-age subjects; this is sometimes referred to as the Z-score and provides a measure of relative osteopenia. The other method is to compare a woman's bone density with the mean and

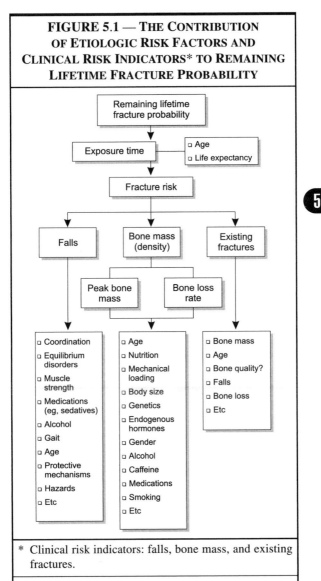

FIGURE 5.1 — THE CONTRIBUTION OF ETIOLOGIC RISK FACTORS AND CLINICAL RISK INDICATORS* TO REMAINING LIFETIME FRACTURE PROBABILITY

Remaining lifetime fracture probability

Exposure time
- Age
- Life expectancy

Fracture risk

Falls

Bone mass (density)

Existing fractures

Peak bone mass

Bone loss rate

- Coordination
- Equilibrium disorders
- Muscle strength
- Medications (eg, sedatives)
- Alcohol
- Gait
- Age
- Protective mechanisms
- Hazards
- Etc

- Age
- Nutrition
- Mechanical loading
- Body size
- Genetics
- Endogenous hormones
- Gender
- Alcohol
- Caffeine
- Medications
- Smoking
- Etc

- Bone mass
- Age
- Bone quality?
- Falls
- Bone loss
- Etc

* Clinical risk indicators: falls, bone mass, and existing fractures.

Modified and reproduced with permission from: Wasnich R. *Am J Med.* 1993;95(suppl 5A):6S-10S.

SD of peak adult bone density; this is known as the T-score and provides a measure of absolute osteopenia. The Z-score is more precise in scientific terms, ie, for evaluating correlations with other variables and for characterizing groups of subjects.

Because the T-score, Z-score, and SD are poorly understood by many patients (and physicians), in the author's opinion the percentage of an individual's bone mass relative to the T-score (peak bone mass) should be used to evaluate:

- Current bone density
- Risk for future fracture
- Degree of bone gained or lost in response to treatment.

Bone Mass: What Is Normal?

What is the dividing line between normal and abnormal? Comparing bone density testing with standard radiographs in normal women and women with radiographic osteopenia but no fractures (prefracture osteoporosis), researchers determined that the bone density in the lumbar spine of prefracture women is 19% less than in a healthy, younger population. Other researchers working independently established that women are at risk for fracture when their bone mass in a given area is reduced by 20% to 30% or more compared with their peak bone mass (35 to 40 years of age). In summary, 80% of peak bone mass (2 SD below the mean) is a practical dividing line between normal bone mass and osteopenia, irrespective of the patient's age. This is a conservative estimate because in most studies a decrease of 1 SD in bone mass is associated with a 50% to 150% increase in the incidence of fractures. Table 5.2 shows a practical, *but not prospectively validated*, classification of degrees of osteopenia.

TABLE 5.2 — CLASSIFICATION OF DEGREES OF OSTEOPENIA		
Bone Mineral Density	**Standard Deviation**	**Degree of Osteopenia**
Peak Bone Mass	*< Young Adult*	*Clinical Staging*
80% to 90%	1 to 2	Mild
70% to 80%	2 to 3	Moderate
<70%	>3	Marked

Another meaningful way of quantifying the significance of low bone mass is to inform patients that:

- A 1-SD decrease in lumbar spine BMD increases the risk for future fracture comparable to a 17-year increase in age
- A 1-SD decrease in femoral BMD is comparable to a 13- to 14-year increase in age concerning the risk of hip fracture.

According to the World Health Organization definition, *a bone density value of -2.5 SD below young adult is diagnostic of osteoporosis.*

Technology Available

To be cost-effective, bone densitometry must be affordable and the equipment must be readily accessible to the public. Long-available technology is not in general use because some test costs are not reimbursed by insurance and because of earlier concerns about the validity and clinical applicability of bone mass measurements. Table 5.3 summarizes characteristics of bone mass measurement techniques, including:

- Precision (reliability of the method for repeated tests)

TABLE 5.3 — TECHNIQUES FOR THE MEASUREMENT OF BONE MASS

Technique	Site	Precision (%)	Accuracy (%)	Examination Time (min)	Radiation Dose* (mrem)	Approximate Cost† ($)
Radiographic absorptiometry	Hand	1 to 2	4	3 to 5	100	75 to 150
Single x-ray absorptiometry	Wrist, heel	1 to 3	5	<1	10 to 20	75 to 150
Dual-energy roentgenogram absorptiometry	Spine, hip, total body	0.5 to 2	3 to 5	3 to 7	1 to 3	150 to 200
Dual-energy x-ray absorptiometry	Finger	<1	1.8	>2	0.00003	?
Quantitative CT	Spine	2 to 5	5 to 20	10 to 15	100 to 1000	150 to 250

* One chest roentgenogram gives a radiation dose of 20 to 50 mrem, a full dental roentgenogram 300 mrem, and an abdominal computed tomography (CT) 1 to 6 mrem.

† Reimbursement approved by the Health Care Financing Administration (HCFA) effective July 1998, is as follows: peripheral densitometry–$41; axial densitometry–$130.

Modified from: Johnson CC Jr, et al. *N Engl J Med.* 1991;324:1105-1109.

- Accuracy (reliability of actual measurements determined by other methods [eg, measurement of ashed weight])
- Time required for examination
- Radiation exposure
- Estimated cost (varies regionally).

Because of the enhanced precision and accuracy of dual-energy x-ray absorptiometry (DEXA), this method has now become the gold standard for bone densitometry. Quantitative computed tomography (CT), with associated radiation exposure, cost, and inaccuracy, is less favored in clinical practice. DEXA provides an accurate measurement of the bone density in the spine and/or hip, enabling the clinician to make objective decisions about the need for hormone therapy, including the type and dose. Repeated measurements at 1-year intervals (and occasionally at 6-month intervals) will quantify the adequacy of treatment and help determine whether the hormone dose or the route of hormone therapy needs to be adjusted. Repeated testing also identifies women with rapid bone loss; this is especially important for women found to have normal bone density on baseline assessment who elect not to receive hormonal or other therapy.

How to Interpret a DEXA Analysis

Although there are three manufacturers of DEXA equipment, the interpretation of the data is similar.

■ **Lumbar Spine Analysis** — (Figure 5.2)
In assessing the quality of the test, the following should be considered:
- Are the vertebrae T12-L5 demonstrated?
- Are the intervertebral spaces clearly defined?
- Is there spinal curvature? If so, has this been compensated for in the analysis?

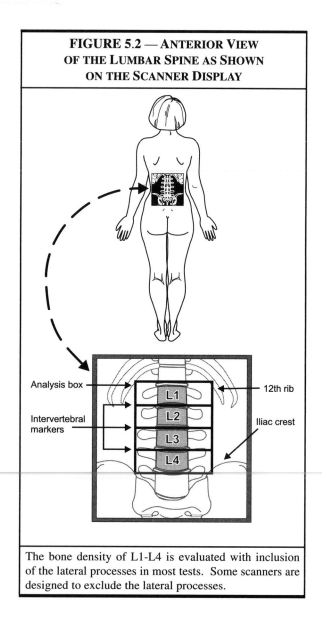

FIGURE 5.2 — ANTERIOR VIEW OF THE LUMBAR SPINE AS SHOWN ON THE SCANNER DISPLAY

Analysis box

12th rib

Intervertebral markers

Iliac crest

L1
L2
L3
L4

The bone density of L1-L4 is evaluated with inclusion of the lateral processes in most tests. Some scanners are designed to exclude the lateral processes.

- Is there a marked difference in the bone density and/or area of vertebrae? If so, this may indicate vertebral fractures and/or ectopic calcification secondary to disk degeneration, arthritis, or a calcified aorta. Check with anteroposterior (AP) and lateral x-ray of the lumbar and thoracic spines.
- Are the patient's demographics correct? This is essential for age-matched comparisons.

- **Interpreting the Data** — (Figures 5.3 and 5.4)
  - Compare the BMD of L2 through L4 with the young adult score (T-score) and the value for age-matched subjects (Z-score).
  - Note the lowest BMD in L1 through L4. Compare with the patient's corresponding young adult value and age-matched values.
  - Note SD below young adult value for each of the above. For every SD below young adult normal, the future risk for fracture increases by 100% to 200%.
  - For patients with moderate to severe osteopenia, take anterior, posterior, and lateral roentgenograms of T4 through L5.
  - Use the data obtained to:
    - Quantify the extent of the condition
    - Decide on appropriate therapy
    - Determine frequency of repeat testing.
  - Monitor response to treatment, using BMD of L2-L4 and the vertebra with the lowest BMD as the marker or denominator.

- **Femoral (Hip) Analysis**
  Three areas of interest are shown in Figure 5.5:
  - Ward's triangle (square box)
  - Femoral neck (area in rectangle)
  - Trochanter.

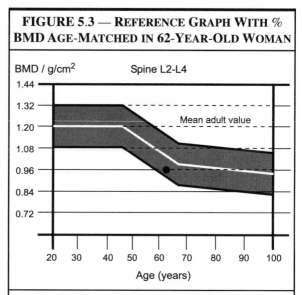

**FIGURE 5.3 — REFERENCE GRAPH WITH %
BMD AGE-MATCHED IN 62-YEAR-OLD WOMAN**

Reference graph with % age-matched (62-year-old). The
example above shows the bone mineral density (BMD)
of a woman age 62 that is 2 standard deviation (SD) below her mean young adult value but is within the limits
of the age-matched regression bar. This shows that while
the patient's BMD is below the mean young adult value,
her low BMD value is "normal" for her age. Shaded area
represents the change in the BMD with age (mean ± 1
SD). Each horizontal bar is equal to 1 SD below mean
peak young adult value.

Modified and reproduced with permission from: Mazess RB.
The Lunar Manual. Madison, Wis: The Lunar Corporation.

■ **Interpreting the Data**

- The type of bone in the femoral neck is primarily cortical; Ward's triangle is a composite of
  cortical and trabecular bone. In the author's experience, the BMD in this area correlates well
  with the BMD in the lumbar spine and ultradistal radius. This was confirmed in a large
  cross-sectional study.

78

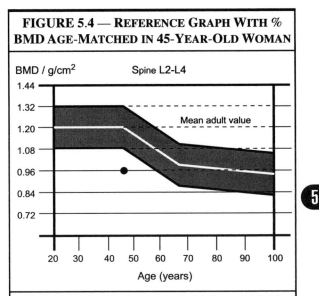

**FIGURE 5.4 — REFERENCE GRAPH WITH %
BMD AGE-MATCHED IN 45-YEAR-OLD WOMAN**

Reference graph with % age-matched (45-year-old). The above figure shows the bone mineral density (BMD) of a 45-year-old patient who has the same BMD value (0.96 g/cm^2) as the 62-year-old shown in Figure 5.3. Unlike the 62-year-old patient, who is above the regression bar, the 45-year-old patient is well below the age-matched regression bar. Shaded area represents the change in the bone mineral density with age (mean ± 1 standard deviation [SD]). Each horizontal bar is equal to 1 SD below mean peak young adult value.

Modified and reproduced with permission from: Mazess RB. *The Lunar Manual*. Madison, Wis: The Lunar Corporation.

- As with the lumbar spine, comparisons of BMD in the above regions are made with the young adult score (T-score) and that of an age-matched subject (Z-score).
- For every SD below young adult normal, the future risk for fracture increases by 100% to 200%.

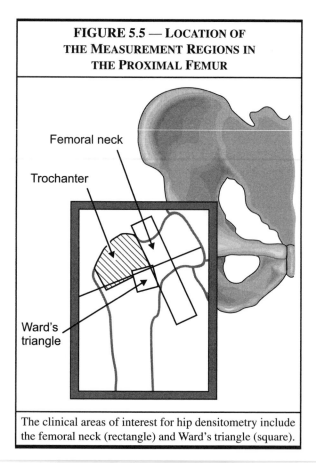

FIGURE 5.5 — LOCATION OF THE MEASUREMENT REGIONS IN THE PROXIMAL FEMUR

Femoral neck

Trochanter

Ward's triangle

The clinical areas of interest for hip densitometry include the femoral neck (rectangle) and Ward's triangle (square).

- Use the data to quantify the degree of osteopenia in the hip and, by repeated testing, the clinical response to treatment.

■ Reference Values

The reference populations are based on studies of healthy subjects without metabolic bone disease or symptomatic or asymptomatic fractures who are not taking medications known to impact on bone physiology. Note: T-scores are calculated from the manufacturers' healthy white young adult reference data bases and may vary according to the instrument used. Adjustments are made for:

- *Age*: For example, "young adult" refers to women between 20 and 39 years of age
- *Ethnic origin*: Black population values are typically 6% greater than those for whites
- *Nationality*: The reference data for Japanese, French, and other nationalities are slightly lower than for white women in the United States
- *Weight*: Heavier patients have higher BMD values and lighter patients lower values than the normal population has. Studies have shown that a 1-kg difference in body weight above or below the norm is associated with a 0.004-g/cm^2 change in the lumbar spine and a 0.003-g/cm^2 change in the femur (femoral neck and Ward's triangle).

The program is adjusted to increase or decrease above the mean, depending on the patient's weight. The mean weight for white women in the United States in the Lunar Data Base is 65 kg. *The program affects the age-matched values only; the weight adjustment does not affect the percentage compared to young adult values.*

Adjustments should be made for patients above or below the mean:

- AP spine: Adjust for women weighing below or above 35 kg and 70 kg, respectively
- Femur: Adjust for weights below or above 35 kg and 100 kg, respectively.

■ Quality Assurance

The DEXA scanner needs to be calibrated on a daily basis according to the manufacturers' internal standard to ensure that:

- The detector peak test (which assesses the system's photon-counting electronics) is within 50 U of the previous peak setting
- Each functional measurement (performed on a spine phantom) must receive a passing evaluation
- The standard values must have a percentage CV of 2.00 or less. Mean values must not deviate from the expected value by >2.5%.

Screening for Osteoporosis

The role of screening for osteoporosis is less clear. We have reported that the bone mineral content of the entire skeleton decreases as a function of age and number of years after menopause, in much the same way as bone mineral is lost from localized areas in the axial and appendicular skeleton. This conclusion has been confirmed by other studies. In our laboratory, bone density of the distal radius measured by single-photon absorptiometry (SPA) correlates well with total bone density ($r = 0.80$; $P < 0.0001$). Others have shown a correlation of $r = 0.6$ between appendicular skeletal sites (distal radius, phalanx, and calcaneus) and spine and hip measurements. We were able to classify correctly 86.3% of 307 untreated women who underwent both SPA and total-body dual-photon absorptiometry (DPA). Only 7.8% of osteopenic women were incorrectly classified as being normal; 5.9% were false-positives (Tesar R, Notelovitz M, unpublished data). In the recent National Osteoporosis Risk Assessment (NORA) study, almost half of the postmenopausal women (none of whom were on antiresorptive therapy, except estrogen) had untested low BMD, including 7% with osteoporosis.

Peripheral tests cannot define the maximal site of osteopenia. More specific analysis of the spine and hip using DEXA is needed. The reason is straightforward:

some patients have generalized osteopenia, whereas others have regionally reduced bone mass in either the spine or hip. Also, the T-scores at different skeletal sites vary greatly. Thus, much like Pap smear screening for cervical cancer, the main purpose of the screening test is to classify individuals into one of three categories:

- Normal
- Abnormal
- Possibly abnormal.

Further testing yields the diagnosis. Figure 5.6, a screening tool based on the author's clinical practice, is one method of cost-effectively monitoring women at risk for osteoporosis.

The role of screening for osteoporosis is still being debated. In 1988, a published review concluded "single-photon absorptiometry of the forearm will become the standard first-line procedure in population screening and in the diagnosis of osteoporosis." SPA has now been replaced with peripheral DEXA testing (SPX). This is accurate for women below the age of 60 when osteopenia of the distal radius correlates well with bone mineral deficiency elsewhere (Figure 5.7). In women over the age of 70, peripheral densitometry tends to overdiagnose axial osteopenia.

Figure 5.8 shows the printout of a distal radius and ulna analyzed on a Lunar DEXA. Based on personal experience (unpublished data), the BMD of the distal radius is a more specific and sensitive indicator of skeletal osteopenia than the BMD of the ulna. In the author's practice, only the distal radius value is measured and compared with young adult and age-matched reference scales. A BMD <80% of the young adult score justifies testing of the spine and the hip in an attempt to define the site of maximal osteopenia.

Other researchers have suggested that a finger or forearm T-score at –3.5 SD (65% of peak adult bone

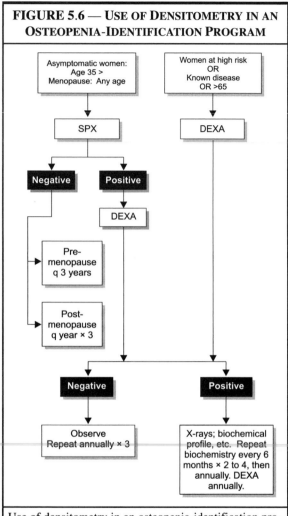

FIGURE 5.6 — USE OF DENSITOMETRY IN AN OSTEOPENIA-IDENTIFICATION PROGRAM

Use of densitometry in an osteopenia-identification program. SPX, rectilinear far distal and proximal dual-energy x-ray absorptiometry of radius; DEXA, dual-energy roentgenographic absorptiometry of L1-L4 and of the proximal femur.

84

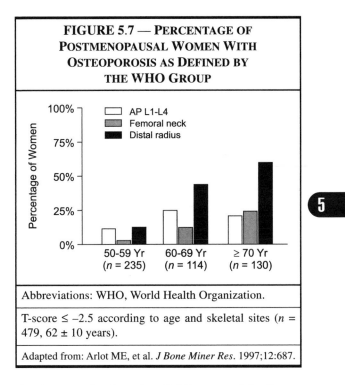

FIGURE 5.7 — PERCENTAGE OF POSTMENOPAUSAL WOMEN WITH OSTEOPOROSIS AS DEFINED BY THE WHO GROUP

Abbreviations: WHO, World Health Organization.

T-score ≤ –2.5 according to age and skeletal sites ($n = 479$, 62 ± 10 years).

Adapted from: Arlot ME, et al. *J Bone Miner Res*. 1997;12:687.

density) is reflective of a –2.5 T-score of the femur. There are a number of instruments based on single-energy x-ray absorptiometry (SXA) technology that measure the BMD of the finger, wrist, and calcaneus. Each method has its own merit; details should be obtained from the respective manufacturers, with particular attention paid to the precision/accuracy of the instrument and its correlation with axial densitometry.

At What Age Should Women Be Screened for Osteoporosis?

The older the individual at the time of screening, the greater the likelihood of detecting low BMD and

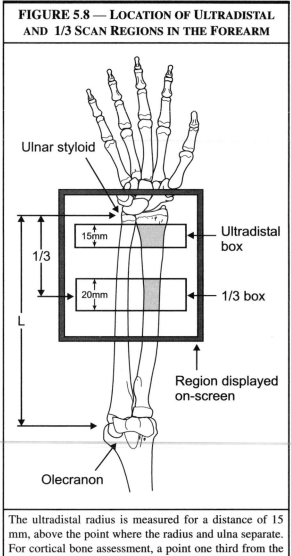

FIGURE 5.8 — LOCATION OF ULTRADISTAL AND 1/3 SCAN REGIONS IN THE FOREARM

Ulnar styloid

15mm

1/3

20mm

Ultradistal box

1/3 box

L

Region displayed on-screen

Olecranon

The ultradistal radius is measured for a distance of 15 mm, above the point where the radius and ulna separate. For cortical bone assessment, a point one third from the styloid process to the olecranon is chosen.

FIGURE 5.9 — RADIOGRAPH OF
THE HAND WITH AN ALUMINUM ALLOY
REFERENCE WEDGE

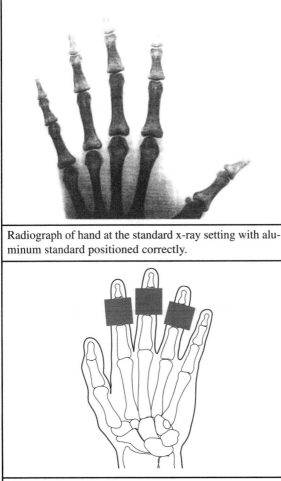

Radiograph of hand at the standard x-ray setting with aluminum standard positioned correctly.

Diagram demonstrating phalangeal scan zones.

Vogt FB, et al. *Am J Roentgenol Radium Ther Nucl Med.* 1969; 105:870-876.

osteoporosis. However, the objective of screening for osteoporosis is to *prevent* its development, and therefore screening should commence at a much younger age. Absent specific clinical indications for early testing, we recommend that women (white, Asian, and Hispanic) consider having their first peripheral bone density test between the ages of 35 and 40. It is at this stage that bone remodeling–associated bone loss accelerates. Diagnosis of osteopenia at this age allows for 10 to 15 years of preventive therapy (including oral contraceptive use) prior to menopause. The first bone density test can be conveniently coordinated with the patient's baseline mammogram.

Radiographic Absorptiometry

Radiographic absorptiometry (RA) determines bone density through computerized analysis of hand radiographs taken by standard diagnostic roentgenographic equipment. In its current form, RA has proved to be a practical, inexpensive, and rapid way to determine BMD:

- Radiographs are taken of the hand together with an aluminum alloy reference wedge (Figure 5.9).
- The developed films are sent to a central laboratory where they are digitized by a high-resolution imaging system.
- A computer analyzes the wedge image and calculates how the optical density of the film is related to the bone mass and wedge imaged on the radiograph. This relationship differs for each film and takes into account film speed, x-ray intensity, and the film processing effects.
- The bone mineral mass of the phalanges is determined and corrections included for bending and rotation of the phalanges and other effects.
- The results are given in arbitrary units, with dimensions of mineral mass per unit volume, and

graphically related to male and female reference norms.

A standard RA assay utilizes two views taken at different radiographic settings, which are analyzed independently and checked for agreement. The radiation exposure from RA (100 mrem) is lower than that of quantitative CT but higher than that of DEXA. However, RA exposes only the hand, not the central body. The internal organ dose for RA is quite low (approximately 1 microsievert) and is approximately equal to that of other densitometry techniques.

In summary:
- RA is a low-cost technique, potentially available at any radiographic facility.
- RA measures both trabecular and cortical bone.
- Recent studies have shown that RA:
  - Is significantly correlated with other standard methods of bone densitometry
  - Has high sensitivity in predicting low bone mass of the lumbar spine and femoral neck (90% and 82%, respectively)
  - Has excellent precision (CV = 0.63% for BMD) and accuracy.

Irrespective of the patient's age, clinical decisions should be based on the individual's value in relationship to peak adult bone mass.

The major disadvantage of RA is the paucity of facilities to process and interpret the x-rays.

Quantitative Bone Ultrasound

The Food and Drug Administration has approved ultrasonometry of bone as a predictive device of osteoporosis and related fractures. Three instruments are available in the United States:
- Lunar Achilles +

- Hologic Sahara
- Myriad Sound-Scan.

As with DEXA technology, key issues in the clinical utility of these instruments is the reproducibility and precision of the measurements. The technology is based on the alteration of the shape, intensity, and speed of sound as it traverses a bony point of interest. This is quantified and serves as a qualitative measurement of the physical and mechanical property of bone, characterized by two measures:

- Speed of sound through bone (ultrasound transit velocity [SOS])
- Attenuation of sound as it passes through bone (broadband ultrasound attenuation [BUA]).

In addition, some instruments (Sahara and Achilles) calculate measures of BUA and SOS to formulate a clinical index (quantitative ultrasound index [QUI]), usually referred to as stiffness.

The site measured (calcaneus; middle third of anterior tibia) and the method of coupling (water or ultrasound gel) vary. A new multi-site assessment of bone ultrasound using ultrasound critical angle reflectometry (UCR) is being evaluated.

Recent studies have shown that quantitative ultrasound (QUS) of the calcaneus is a predictor of hip fracture risk that is independent of femoral BMD. It is currently accepted that 10% to 30% QUS reports are influenced by the microarchitecture of bone, the mineral constituents of bone matrix, and the elastic modulus (and hence the strength) of bone. The remainder is accounted for by the BMD of bone. There is, however, no consensus on this point.

Cross-sectional and longitudinal studies have demonstrated—as with BMD—a decrease in both SOS and BUA measures after menopause and that this technology can discriminate (fairly accurately) between

90

normal and osteoporotic subjects. For every standard deviation decrease in BUA of the calcaneus, the risk of hip fracture increases twofold, a result identical to that with equivalent decrease in hip BMD.

Thus QUS may be a useful measure of bone strength and of additional value in quantifying an individual's actual risk for fracture, for example, in individuals with relatively normal BMD but low QUS. Recent studies have shown that although QUS and BMD have and share certain heritable traits, specific genes appear to have greater effects than shared genes in each trait. Ultrasound is not recommended at this time for the monitoring of treatment.

Newer Technology

The present DEXA technology measures two different components by separating bone mineral from lean soft tissue. This assumes that there is a constant relationship between lean soft tissue and adipose tissue. Unfortunately, this simplification may result in significant measurement errors. A new technology incorporates laser technology to a dual-energy x-ray source. This simple solution allows for the measurement of three different components (bone mineral, lean soft tissue, and adipose tissue, including yellow bone marrow) instead of the usual two (Figure 5.10).

Variations of adipose tissue no longer create errors in true bone density measurements. As a result, the monitors using this technology (DXL Calscan, manufactured by Demetech AB in Sweden) have an accuracy of 98% (standard error of estimate <2%) and a measurement coefficient of <1.2% *in vivo* and 0.5% *in vitro*. Precision of this degree allows for distinguishing minor changes in BMD, and therefore this technology is useful for monitoring of treatment. The instrument, which measures the BMD of the calcaneus, has an internal phantom that automatically calibrates

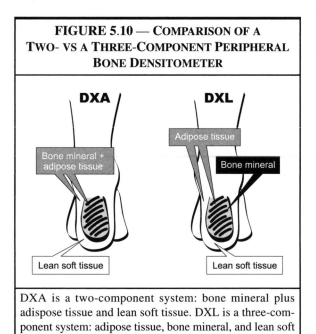

FIGURE 5.10 — COMPARISON OF A TWO- VS A THREE-COMPONENT PERIPHERAL BONE DENSITOMETER

DXA is a two-component system: bone mineral plus adispose tissue and lean soft tissue. DXL is a three-component system: adipose tissue, bone mineral, and lean soft tissue.

the instrument before each new patient. The DXL Calscan also has an automatic region of interest, which makes the results operator-independent by defining the ideal scanning site on the initial and subsequent measurements. Scanning of the heel takes <1 minute. As with other BMD scanners, T- and Z-scores are available for clinical interpretation of individual results.

SUGGESTED READING

Arlot ME, Sornay-Rendu E, Garnero P, Vey-Marty B, Delmas PD. Apparent pre- and postmenopausal bone loss evaluated by DXA at different skeletal sites in women: the OFELY cohort. *J Bone Miner Res.* 1997;12:683-690.

Bauer DC, Glüer CC, Cauley JA, et al. Broadband ultrasound attenuation predicts fractures strongly and independently of densitometry in older women. A prospective study. Study of Osteoporotic Fractures Research Group. *Arch Intern Med.* 1997;157: 629-634.

Binkley NC, Schmeer P, Wasnich RD, Lenchik L. What are the criteria by which a densitometric diagnosis of osteoporosis can be made in males and non-caucasians? *J Clin Densitom.* 2002;5(suppl)S19-S27.

Clinical indications for bone mass measurements. A report from the Scientific Advisory Board of the National Osteoporosis Foundation. *J Bone Miner Res.* 1989;4(suppl 2):1-28.

Cosman F, Herrington B, Himmelstein S, Lindsay R. Radiographic absorptiometry: a simple method for determination of bone mass. *Osteoporos Int.* 1991;2:34-38.

Cummings SR, Black DM, Nevitt MC, et al. Appendicular bone density and age predict hip fracture in women. The Study of Osteoporotic Fractures Research Group. *JAMA.* 1990;263:665-668.

Davis JW, Ross PD, Wasnich RD. Evidence for both generalized and regional low bone mass among elderly women. *J Bone Miner Res.* 1994;9:305-309.

Glüer CC. Quantitative ultrasound techniques for the assessment of osteoporosis: expert agreement on current status. The International Quantitative Ultrasound Consensus Group. *J Bone Miner Res.* 1997;12:1280-1288.

Gotfredsen A, Nilas L, Riis BJ, Thomsen K, Christiansen C. Bone changes occurring spontaneously and caused by estrogen in early postmenopausal women: a local or generalised phenomenon? *Br Med J.* 1986;292:1098-1100.

5

Hamdy RC, Petak SM, Lenchik L. Which central dual x-ray absorptiometry skeletal sites and regions of interest should be used to determine the diagnosis of osetoporosis? *J Clin Densitom.* 2002;5(suppl)S11-S17.

Hodsman AB. Bone mineral density T-scores: assessing the risk. *Clin Invest Med.* 1998;21:94-96.

Howard GM, Nguyen TV, Harris M, Kelly PJ, Eisman JA. Genetic and environmental contributions to the association between quantitative ultrasound and bone mineral density measurements: a twin study. *J Bone Miner Res.* 1998;13:1318-1327.

Hui SL, Slemenda CW, Johnston CC Jr. Age and bone mass as predictors of fracture in a prospective study. *J Clin Invest.* 1988;81:1804-1809.

Johnston CC Jr, Slemenda CW, Melton LJ III. Clinical use of bone densitometry. *N Engl J Med.* 1991;324:1105-1109.

Kanis JA. Diagnosis of osteoporosis and assessment of fracture risk. *Lancet.* 2002;359:1929-1936.

Lenchik L, Kiebzak GM, Blunt BA. What is the role of serial bone mineral density measurements in patient management? *J Clin Densitom.* 2002;5(suppl)S29-S38.

Lindsay R, Silverman SL, Cooper C, et al. Risk of new vertebral fracture in the year following a fracture. *JAMA.* 2001;285:320-323.

Looker AC, Beck TJ, Orwoll ES. Does body size account for gender differences in femur bone density and geometry? *J Bone Miner Res.* 2001;16:1291-1299.

Mazess RB. *The Lunar Manual.* Madison, Wis: The Lunar Corporation.

Mazess RB, Barden H, Ettinger M, Schultz E. Bone density of the radius, spine, and proximal femur in osteoporosis. *J Bone Miner Res.* 1988;3:13-18.

Melton LJ III, Atkinson EJ, O'Fallon WM, Wahner HW, Riggs BL. Long-term fracture prediction by bone mineral assessed at different skeletal sites. *J Bone Miner Res.* 1993;8:1227-1233.

Melton LJ III, Eddy DM, Johnston CC Jr. Screening for osteoporosis. *Ann Intern Med*. 1990;112:516-528.

Melton LJ III, Chao EY, Lane J. Biomechanical aspects of fractures. In: Riggs BL, Melton LJ III, eds. *Osteoporosis: Etiology, Diagnosis and Management*. New York, NY: Raven Press; 1988: 111-121.

Naessen T, Mallmin H, Ljunghall S. Heel ultrasound in women after long-term ERT compared with bone densities in the forearm, spine and hip. *Osteoporos Int*. 1995;5:205-210.

Need AG, Nordin BE. Which bone to measure? *Osteoporos Int*. 1990;1:3-6.

NIH Consensus Development Panel on Osteoporosis Prevention, Diagnosis, and Therapy. Osteoporosis prevention, diagnosis, and therapy. *JAMA*. 2001;285:785-795.

Njeh CF, Gordon CL, Hans D, et al. The new generation of bone densitometers. *Contemp Obstet Gynecol*. 1998;April:15-40.

Nordin BE, Wishart JM, Horowitz M, Need AG, Bridges A, Bellon M. The relation between forearm and vertebral mineral density and fractures in postmenopausal women. *Bone Miner*. 1988;5:21-33.

Notelovitz M. Post-menopausal osteoporosis. A practical approach to its prevention. *Acta Obstet Gynecol Scand*. 1986;134(suppl):67-80.

Parfitt AM. Interpretation of bone densitometry measurements: disadvantages of a percentage scale and a discussion of some alternatives. *J Bone Miner Res*. 1990;5:537-540.

Riggs BL, Melton LJ III. Involutional osteoporosis. *N Engl J Med*. 1986;314:1676-1686.

Ross PD, Wasnich RD, Vogel JM. Detection of prefracture spinal osteoporosis using bone mineral absorptiometry. *J Bone Miner Res*. 1988;3:1-11.

Sturtridge W, Lentle B, Hanley DA. Prevention and management of osteoporosis: consensus statements from the Scientific Advisory Board of the Osteoporosis Society of Canada. 2. The use of bone density measurement in the diagnosis and management of osteoporosis. *CMAJ*. 1996;155:924-929.

5

Tesar R, Notelovitz M. Comparisons of bone mineral results using single and dual-photon absorptiometry in osteoporosis. In: Christiansen C, Arnaud CD, Nordin BED, et al, eds. *Osteoporosis, 1983*. Copenhagen, Denmark: Glostrup Hospital; 1983:213-225.

Vogt FB, Meharg LS, Mack PB. Use of a digital computer in the measurement of roentgenographic bone density. *Am J Roentgenol Radium Ther Nucl Med*. 1969;105:870-876.

Wasnich R. Bone mass measurement: prediction of risk. *Am J Med*. 1993;95(suppl 5A):6S-10S.

Wasnich RD, Ross PD, Heilbrun LK, Vogel JM. Prediction of postmenopausal fracture risk with use of bone mineral measurements. *Am J Obstet Gynecol*. 1985;153:745-751.

6 Diagnosing Osteoporosis

Vertebral Fractures

Osteoporosis is a skeletal disease characterized by low bone mass and microarchitectural deterioration of bone tissue, leading to enhanced bone fragility and a consequent increase in fracture risk. It accounts for approximately 117 fractures per 100,000 person-years. Vertebral fractures, which are frequently asymptomatic, usually occur within 15 to 20 years of menopause. Lateral roentgenograms of the thoracic and lumbar spine not only help to identify these fractures but also quantify the biomechanical significance of reduced bone mass.

Osteopenia, bone mineral deficiency in the absence of fracture, is an indirect indicator of the bone's structural integrity. Compared with osteoporosis, osteopenia has greater treatment potential, ie, it is possible to improve bone mass and associated bone strength, as well as prevent fractures. Combined information about low bone mass and a prevalent (existing) fracture is better for predicting new fractures than either variable alone.

In a recent study, the presence of one or more prevalent vertebral fractures at baseline increased the risk of further fracture fivefold during the first year of observation compared with those subjects who were fracture free at baseline (relative risk [RR] 5:1) (Figure 6.1).

Three degrees of vertebral deformation are recognized:
- End-plate deformity

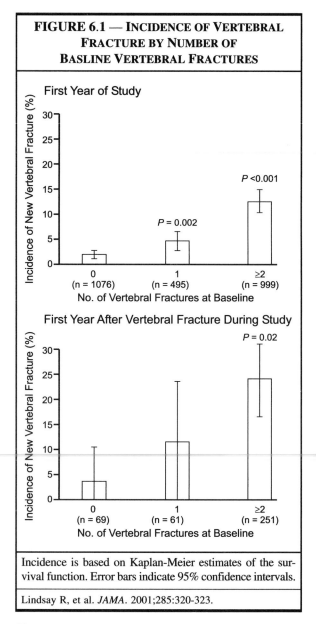

FIGURE 6.1 — INCIDENCE OF VERTEBRAL FRACTURE BY NUMBER OF BASLINE VERTEBRAL FRACTURES

Incidence is based on Kaplan-Meier estimates of the survival function. Error bars indicate 95% confidence intervals.

Lindsay R, et al. *JAMA*. 2001;285:320-323.

- Anterior wedge deformity
- Compression deformity.

A vertebral deformation score has been proposed that can be used in longitudinal studies to quantify objectively the progress of the condition and/or response to treatment. At least 14 vertebrae (T4 through L4) should be roentgenographed. The anterior, middle, and posterior heights of the vertebrae are measured, and the fracture can be then classified as follows:

- *Mildly depressed (grade 1)*: 20% to 25% decrease in anterior, middle, and/or posterior height and/or reduction in 10% to 20% of the area
- *Moderately deformed (grade 2)*: 25% to 40% reduction in the height and/or a reduction in area of 20% to 40%
- *Severely deformed (grade 3)*: 40% reduction in any height and area.

Using the above criteria, clinicians are frequently surprised to find that many patients who seem to have "obvious" osteoporosis and clinically apparent dorsal kyphosis have normal roentgenograms. Scheuermann's kyphosis, for example, is associated with a relatively sharp curvature of the dorsal spine but with normal vertebral bodies and bone mineral. Roentgenograms are relatively crude indices of fracture and may obscure latent fracture. Also, there are no currently available practical methods of assessing microfractures and/or disruption of the microarchitecture of the plates in vertebral bone, although a newer MRI-based technology may soon resolve this clinical need.

Supine lateral dual-energy x-ray absorptiometry (DEXA) is a promising technique and is a better index of vertebral bone strength and the potential risk for future fracture than anterior-posterior DEXA measurement and lateral roentgenograms. However, the reliability of the technique in clinical practice is limited by the ability to clearly define only L3, L4, and sometimes L2. Most osteoporotic fractures occur above this level. Difficulty with patient positioning is also a potential limiting factor, although this disadvantage has been resolved by improved positioning technology in some of the newer densitometers.

Roentgenograms serve three useful clinical purposes. They can identify disk degeneration and osteoarthritis as causes of back pain and thus indicate a different approach to treatment, and they are helpful in clarifying why some patients with known osteoporosis can have relatively normal bone mineral density (BMD).

Previous microfractures with callous formation artificially increase bone mass measurement, as do degenerative disk disease, osteoarthritis, and calcification of the overlying abdominal aorta. Lateral DEXA analysis may be able to resolve some of these confounding issues (Figure 6.2).

Until recently, prevalent vertebral fractures were considered to be noncorrectable. A new technique—percutaneous vertebral augmentation (PVA)—has been developed with the primary objective of relieving pain and other sequelae of osteoporotic vertebral fractures. Two techniques are available: vertebroplasty and kyphoplasty. Because of the heterogenecity of vertebral compression fractures, morphometry of the affected area(s) is essential.

Hip Fractures

Hip fractures are due to a slow but progressive loss of both cortical and cancellous (trabecular) bone at comparable rates. The bone loss is "silent" and eventually manifests in fractures in individuals over 70 years of age. There is only a weak correlation between vertebral fractures and future hip fracture.

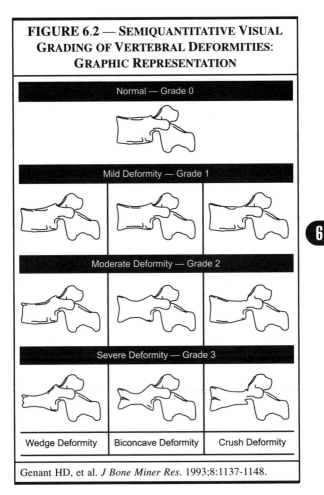

FIGURE 6.2 — SEMIQUANTITATIVE VISUAL GRADING OF VERTEBRAL DEFORMITIES: GRAPHIC REPRESENTATION

Normal — Grade 0

Mild Deformity — Grade 1

Moderate Deformity — Grade 2

Severe Deformity — Grade 3

| Wedge Deformity | Biconcave Deformity | Crush Deformity |

Genant HD, et al. *J Bone Miner Res*. 1993;8:1137-1148.

Dual energy x-ray absorptiometry assessment of the BMD of the femoral neck, Ward's triangle, and, to a lesser extent, the trochanter is a good measure of potential hip fracture.

There are three radiologic measures that are also useful as predictors of hip fracture:

- Singh index

- Femoral neck length
- Femoral width measurements.

■ Singh Index

The trabeculae of the hip are arranged in various groups that reflect the stress across the joint. The most prominent of these stress trabeculae are the vertically oriented principal compressive trabeculae and the more horizontally placed principal tensile trabeculae. There are also secondary trabeculae. The Singh index is based on the integrity of the trabeculae of the principal and secondary tensile and compressive groups.

As bone is lost, the non–stress-bearing trabeculae are absorbed while the stress trabeculae are reinforced and become even more prominent on roentgenogram. The Singh index is a subjective method of quantifying the appearance of the stress trabeculae into various grades according to a set reference of radiographs (Figure 6.3).

More recently, the type of femoral fracture can be predicted by differentiating the BMD of the upper versus the lower femoral neck region. Cervical neck fractures were associated with low BMD of the upper femoral neck region; trochanteric fractures had low BMD in both areas. This correlates with the difference in the biomechanical strength of bone associated with compressive (lower femoral neck) and tensile (upper femoral neck) stress on the hip.

■ Femoral Neck Length

Increasing femoral neck length (hip axial length [HAL]) raises the risk for hip fracture and may be independent of bone mass assessment of the hip in the femoral neck but not in trochanteric fractures. This may account for the lower risk of hip fracture in Asian women, who characteristically have shorter HAL. Software to measure HAL is now available.

FIGURE 6.3— DIAGRAMMATIC REPRESENTATION OF THE SINGH INDEX

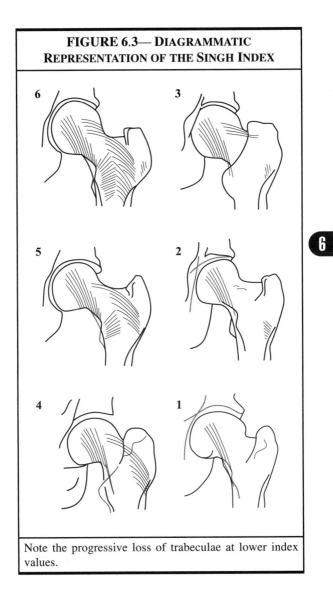

Note the progressive loss of trabeculae at lower index values.

■ Femoral Width Measurements

The measurement of various femoral bone widths, as illustrated in Figure 6.4, is predictive of hip fractures in combination with measurement of the bone density of the hip. To standardize the radiograph, patients are kept supine with their feet taped at a 15° to

---

FIGURE 6.4 — FEMORAL AND PELVIC BONES: PLACEMENT OF SELECTED RADIOGRAPHIC MEASUREMENTS

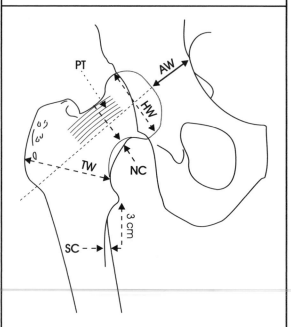

Radiographic Measurements: The thickness of the medial shaft cortex (SC) 3 cm below the lesser trochanter; the thickness of the medial cortex at the center of the femoral neck (NC); the femoral head width (HW), the intertrochanteric region width (TW), and acetabular bone width (AW). The region of the principal tensile (PT) group of trabeculae is marked.

30° internal rotation using a 40-inch focal radiograph distance, with the beam centered on the pubic symphysis. There are limitations to this technique, and standardization is necessary to account for variations in:

- Patient size
- Positioning (including repositioning with follow-up exam)
- Subjective assessment by the radiologist
- Precise measurement
- Pelvic radiation: 1140 Sv vs 1 Sv for DEXA test of the hip.

In the author's opinion, pelvic radiographs may help to quantify the significance of the bone strength in patients with low bone density measurements of the hip. Radiologic abnormalities indicative of a decrease in the tensile strength of the bone (quality), together with some of the previously noted anatomic and geometric factors, may be predictive of an increased risk of future fracture over and above that associated with low BMD.

For example, the lower risk of femoral fracture in men appears to be more related to biomechanical factors rather than a real BMD-increased subperiosteal width, section module, and cortical thickness in the male femoral neck compared with weight-matched women.

Evolving New Technologies

Microarchitectural disruption of the trabecular plates in cancellous bone is a major factor in the etiology of osteoporotic fractures. A new technique, digital topologic analysis (DTA), applied to magnetic resonance microimages of the radius, allows a three-dimensional inspection of the trabecular bone network. The demonstration and quantification of the conversion of trabecular plates to rods and disconnectivity of the trabecula in the distal radius is strongly correlated with the extent of vertebral deformities. In some instances, the degree of microarchitectural disruption exceed that of changes in bone density and/or bone volume (Figure 6.5).

Figure 6.5 represents a way of quantifying the network erosion of trabeculae from osteoclastic action. The process is predominant during aging and in individuals with osteoporosis, and it is the end result of the conversion of trabecular plates to rods.

Evaluating Secondary Causes of Osteoporosis

Most patients with documented osteoporosis do not have endocrinopathies that account for their bone mineral deficiency. When this is suspected on clinical grounds or when patients are nonresponsive to appropriate treatment (eg, hormone therapy), tests of thyroid, parathyroid, and adrenal functions are warranted. Patients suspected of osteomalacia and neoplastic disease need specialized and specific testing. A useful screen for multiple myeloma (which causes spontaneous vertebral fractures and back pain) is the sedimentation rate.

SUGGESTED READING

Black DM, Cummings SR, Stone K, Hudes E, Palermo L, Steiger P. A new approach to defining normal vertebral dimensions. *J Bone Miner Res.* 1991;6:883-892.

Cummings SR, Cauley JA, Palermo L, et al. Racial differences in hip axis lengths might explain racial differences in rates of hip fracture. Study of Osteoporotic Fractures Research Group. *Osteoporos Int.* 1994;4:226-229.

FIGURE 6.5 — SPINE, CROSS-SECTIONAL RADIUS, AND VIRTUAL CORE 3D SURFACE PROJECTIONS

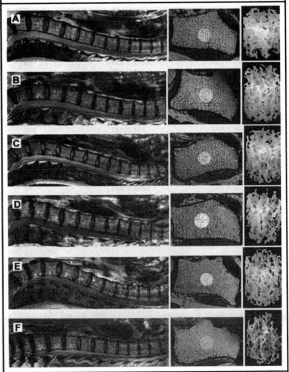

Spine, cross-sectional radius, and virtual core 3D surface projections from region of interest indicated (left, center, and right) for (A-C) three subjects without spinal deformities and (D-F) three with deformities. Dual-energy x-ray absorptiometry for bone mass index (DXA-BMD) (L2-L4) indicated that subjects in panels A and C were normal, in panels D-F were osteopenic, and in panel B was osteoporotic. Patients with vertebral fractures had high erosion index values unlike their normal peers.

Wehrli FW, et al. *J Bone Miner Res.* 2001;16:1520-1531.

Duboeuf F, Hans D, Schott AM, et al. Different morphometric and densitometric parameters predict cervical and trochanteric hip fracture: the EPIDOS Study. *J Bone Miner Res.* 1997;12:1895-1902.

Eastell R, Cedel SL, Wahner HW, Riggs BL, Melton LJ III. Classification of vertebral fractures. *J Bone Miner Res.* 1991;6:207-215.

Faulkner KG, Cummings SR, Black D, Palermo L, Glüer CC, Genant HK. Simple measurement of femoral geometry predicts hip fracture: the study of osteoporotic fractures. *J Bone Miner Res.* 1993;8:1211-1217.

Faulkner KG, Glüer CC, Palermo L, et al. Geometric measurements from dual x-ray absorptiometry scans predict hip fracture. *J Bone Miner Res.* 1993;7(suppl 1):98.

Genant HK, Wu CY, van Kuijk C, Nevitt MC. Vertebral fracture assessment using a semiquantitative technique. *J Bone Miner Res.* 1993;8:1137-1148.

Glüer CC, Cummings SR, Pressman A, et al. Prediction of hip fractures from pelvic radiographs: the study of osteoporotic fractures. The Study of Osteoporotic Fractures Research Group. *J Bone Miner Res.* 1994;9:671-677.

Myers BS, Arbogast KB, Lobaugh B, Harper KD, Richardson WJ, Drezner MK. Improved assessment of lumbar vertebral body strength using supine lateral dual-energy x-ray absorptiometry. *J Bone Miner Res.* 1994;9:687-693.

Ross PD, Davis JW, Epstein RS, Wasnich RD. Pre-existing fractures and bone mass predict vertebral fracture incidence in women. *Ann Intern Med.* 1991;114:919-923.

Sauer P, Leidig G, Minne HW, et al. Spine deformity index (SDI) versus other objective procedures of vertebral fracture identification in patients with osteoporosis: a comparative study. *J Bone Miner Res.* 1991;6:227-238.

7 Evaluating Bone Remodeling

Bone mass measurement and roentgenograms are relatively static indicators of bone health and do not reflect the activity of the bone-remodeling cycle. As noted previously, bone formation is initiated by activation of osteoclasts, whose primary function is to remove old bone and to set the stage for osteoblasts to lay down osteoid, which is mineralized to form new and structurally stronger bone.

Markers of Bone Formation

A number of biochemical markers have been identified, some of which are currently available and useful in clinical practice.

■ Bone-Specific Serum Alkaline Phosphatase Activity

This is the most accurate and practical marker of bone formation and is reflective of osteoblast function. It is a useful measure (especially in combination with some of the other markers) of activation of the bone remodeling cycle. As such, it can be used as a measure of clinical response in patients being treated for conditions with known high bone mineral–turnover loss (eg, hyperthyroidism) and in patients with low bone formation rates on some treatments (eg, androgens and ?intermittent parathyroid hormone [PTH]). Presence of an elevated or low serum alkaline phosphatase level may explain a patient's clinical response or failure to respond, respectively.

The clinician should know the laboratory's reference values and ensure that repeat tests use the same assay and are performed in the same laboratory; values do not need to be out of the reference range. Levels of alkaline phosphatase in the high or low normal range should be viewed as relative measures of turnover. Tests should be repeated at 6-month intervals to monitor change over time and to relate levels to the patient's clinical response. The bone-specific alkaline phosphatase isoenzyme test (using monoclonal antibodies) must be differentiated from the nonspecific assay routinely performed as part of liver function tests. This assay lacks sensitivity and specificity to bone and may be indicative of other metabolic activity or pathology.

■ Serum Osteocalcin or Bone GLA-Protein

This protein is specific to bone and related tissues. Although its true function is unknown, osteocalcin (synthesized by osteoblasts) can be used as a marker of bone mineral metabolism. Osteocalcin secretion is circadian, with the peak level at 4 AM and the nadir at 5 PM. This cyclic activity is said to reflect an increase of bone turnover at night. The difference between peak and trough values is approximately 15%. Although useful in clinical research, the role of bone GLA-protein in clinical practice is yet to be defined.

■ Other Markers

A potentially important marker is one of the procollagen I extension peptides, the aminoterminal derivative (P coll I-N), which is a by-product of the extracellular metabolism of type I collagen. These peptides circulate in blood and, as such, may be useful as a systemic measure of bone collagen, the predominant component of bone matrix. This would add an important component to the assessment of treatment efficacy because most currently available techniques reflect bone mineral metabolism alone.

Two other bone proteins secreted by osteoblasts are osteonectin and bone sialoprotein II. Both proteins are also produced by platelets and, therefore, more specific monoclonal antibodies must be developed before the test can be specific enough for clinical use.

Markers of Bone Resorption

■ Urinary Calcium Excretion

The most useful marker of bone mineral loss is the 24-hour excretion rate of calcium or, more conveniently, the early morning calcium-to-creatinine ratio. The second voided sample of urine after an overnight fast is assayed for calcium and creatinine. If the ratio exceeds 0.16, it is indicative of bone mineral loss. The patient's calcium intake can influence the result and should not exceed 1500 mg/day.

A 24-hour urine collection to assess calcium excretion is inconvenient for the patient, and samples are often incomplete and, therefore, inadequate for assessment. Calcium values in excess of 300 mg/24 hours are indicative of excessive bone mineral mobilization. The author recommends measurement of the urinary calcium–creatine ratio initial assessment, especially if the patient's BMD is reduced. The reason: osteopenia in some women is associated with idiopathic hypercalciuria secondary to reduced renal tubular reabsorption of calcium. This condition is nonresponsive to antiresorptive agents but is corrected by 50 mg hydrochlorothiazide (HCTZ) daily. Long-term treatment with HCTZ is associated with a significant decrease in hip fracture.

■ Urinary Hydroxyproline

This less frequently used marker of resorption reflects the degradation of collagen. Because this is in large measure due to the resorption of bone matrix, the marker complements the urinary calcium excretion test. Unfortunately, since urine hydroxyproline is also derived from the breakdown of collagen in other tissues, its use as a marker of bone resorption is not highly specific. Two additional disadvantages are the cost of the test and the need for the patient to be on a special gelatin-free diet for at least 3 days before the test. Twenty-four hour urine samples are required.

■ Urinary Excretion of Collagen Cross-links

Collagen cross-links are the accepted markers of bone resorption. Two cross-links present in mature collagen, pyridinoline (Pyr) and deoxypyridinoline (dPyr), are found in low concentrations in connective tissue but in higher amounts in type I collagen of bone (Pyr and dPyr) and in type II collagen of cartilage (Pyr only). Both Pyr and dPyr are excreted in bound and free forms and were originally measured by fluorometry. This technology has been replaced by highly specific immunoassays. These assays measure the telopeptide fractions of the type I collagen degradation products in urine, C-carboxytelopeptide (CTx) and N-carboxytelopeptide (NTx).

The urinary levels of the free and bound cross-linked CTx and NTx of type I collagen have been shown to be a sensitive and specific marker of bone resorption. The cross-linked peptides measured in this assay are derived specifically from bone collagen degradation and are not metabolized. Urinary collagen cross-links are significantly increased after menopause and are returned to premenopausal levels by hormone therapy. These tests have been validated for clinical practice and are the best methods of assessing bone matrix metabolism. For example, elderly women with urinary bone resorption markers above the premenopausal upper limit have a twofold increased risk of hip fracture. There is a substantial interindividual and intraindividual variation in the test results due to the diurnal excretion of the collagen by-products and variability in urine dilution. This has been corrected by standardizing the result by correction for creatinine and by collecting samples at a uniform time: second voided sample of urine after an overnight fast. Three commercial preparations are available: urinary type I CTx (CrossLaps; Osteometer Biotech A/S); urinary type I NTx (Ostex International); and urine-free dPyr (Metro Biosystem).

■ Serum Markers of Biochemical Markers

To overcome the inconvenience of having to collect early morning urine samples, serum assays for both the type 1 CTx and the type 1 NTx have been developed. Comparative studies have confirmed the importance of the physiologic diurnal variations of the bone markers in both premenopausal and postmenopausal women. This is due to the increased bone turnover during the night. Although some studies have shown that serum NTx has shown slightly lower variability in results compared with equivalent urine assays, it would appear that patient preparation and timing of the test are what count most. Early morning testing after an overnight fast appears to be essential to minimizing day-to-day variation in test results.

Measurement of urinary cross-links in the afternoon, for example, may underestimate the bone turnover by 30% to 40% compared with an early morning urine sample (Table 7.1).

Clinical Message: The biochemical markers of bone remodeling are an important complement to BMD testing, as they provide a dynamic assessment of current bone turnover to the more static measure of skeletal status provided by BMD. Al-

TABLE 7.1 — BIOCHEMICAL MARKERS OF BONE TURNOVER

Formation	Resorption
Most Efficient Markers	
	Pyr and dPyr collagen cross-links and related peptides
Osteocalcin (BGP)	
Bone alkaline phosphatase	
Other Markers	
Total alkaline phosphatase	Urinary hydroxyproline
Procollagen I extension peptides	Urinary hydroxylysine glycosides
	Plasma tartrate-resistance acid phosphatase

Abbreviations: Pyr, pyridinoline; dPyr, deoxypyridinoline.

though not appropriate for diagnosing osteoporosis, bone markers meet the following important clinical needs:

- The test results differentiate between osteopenia and osteoporosis associated with either high or low turnover bone remodeling. This facilitates the selection of antiresorptive or bone-forming drugs (see Chapter 12).
- Biochemical markers provide rapid assessment of the efficacy of antiresorptive drugs. The values 3 months posttreatment should be decreased by 30% to 50% from baseline. If this is not observed, either the dose or type of drug prescribed needs to be adjusted.
- Bone marker excretion is predictive of the risk of vertebral and hip fracture, independent of BMD measurement. Combining BMD tests with urinary collagen excretion enhances the fracture risk prediction.

Given the need to keep medical costs within affordable limits, the author relies on a combination of the urinary calcium-to-creatinine ratio and the Sequential Multiple Analysis-25 (SMA-25) profile. This profile evaluates non–bone-specific alkaline phosphatase, calcium, and phosphorus and tests of liver and kidney function, all of which have practical implications associated with bone mineral metabolism. To evaluate the bone matrix, the battery of tests should include the assay of serum or urinary NTx type 1 collagen (Osteomark-NTX) or free deoxypyridinoline (Pyrilinks-D).

In untreated osteopenic or osteoporotic women with low or normal collagen excretion, a bone-specific alkaline phosphatase test will identify an underlying osteoblast dysfunction and the need for osteogenic/anabolic bone therapy, eg, androgens, sodium fluoride, or PTH (see Chapter 13).

SUGGESTED READING

Chaki O, Yoshikata I, Kikuchi R, et al. The predictive value of biochemical markers of bone turnover for bone mineral density in postmenopausal Japanese women. *J Bone Miner Res.* 2000;15:1537-1544.

Chapurlat RD, Garnero P, Breart G, Meunier PJ, Delmas PD. Serum type I collagen breakdown product (serum CTX) predicts hip fracture risk in elderly women: The EPIDOS Study. *Bone.* 2000;27:283-286.

Christiansen C, Riis BJ, Rodbro P. Prediction of rapid bone loss in postmenopausal women. *Lancet.* 1987;1:1105-1108.

Delmas PD. Biochemical markers of bone turnover. I: Theoretical considerations and clinical use in osteoporosis. *Am J Med.* 1993;95(suppl 5A):11S-16S.

Delmas PD. Clinical use of biochemical markers of bone remodeling in osteoporosis. In: Christiansen C, Overgaard K, eds. *Osteoporosis 1990.* Copenhagen, Denmark: Osteopress Aps; 1990: 450-458.

Fall PM, Kennedy D, Smith JA, Seibel MJ, Raisz LG. Comparison of serum and urine assays for biochemical markers of bone resorption in postmenopausal women with and without hormone replacement therapy and in men. *Osteoporos Int.* 2000;11:481-485.

Farley SM, Wergedal JE, Smith LC, Lundy MW, Farley JR, Baylink DJ. Fluoride therapy for osteoporosis: characterization of the skeletal response by serial measurements of serum alkaline phosphatase activity. *Metabolism.* 1987;36:211-218.

Looker AC, Bauer DC, Chesnut CH 3rd, et al. Clinical use of biochemical markers of bone remodeling: current status and future directions. *Osteoporos Int.* 2000;11:467-480.

Pyridinium crosslinks as markers of bone resorption. *Lancet.* 1992;340:278-279. Editorial.

Reginster JY, Henrotin Y, Christiansen C, et al. Bone resorption in post-menopausal women with normal and low BMD assessed with biochemical markers specific for telopeptide derived degradation products of collagen type I. *Calcif Tissue Int.* 2001;69:130-137.

Riis BJ. Biochemical markers of bone turnover. II: Diagnosis, prophylaxis, and treatment of osteoporosis. *Am J Med.* 1993;95(suppl 5A):17S-21S.

Rosen HN, Dresner-Pollak R, Moses AC, et al. Specificity of urinary excretion of cross-linked N-telopeptides of type I collagen as a marker of bone turnover. *Calcif Tissue Int.* 1994;54:26-29.

8 Clinical Evaluation of the Musculoskeletal System in Women With Osteoporosis

Women are generally more concerned about spinal than hip fractures. The resulting back pain and disfigurement of vertebral fracture are of great concern to patients and are significant in the subsequent management and rehabilitation of these patients. Rather surprisingly, back pain 12 weeks after the initial postfracture healing phase is usually unrelated to the actual fracture site. This is especially true for patients with persistent pain who are seen some months or years later. Therefore, although bone is the primary site of pathology in osteoporotic subjects, the evaluation of the patient should include systems remote from, yet intimately associated with, the skeleton.

Evaluation of the Patient

■ History

In patients with osteoporosis, such factors as a family history of osteoporosis, the regularity of the menstrual cycle, and the onset of menopause are of minor relevance compared with events surrounding the actual time of fracture and the presence of other factors that could impact on the musculoskeletal system.

Researchers have documented a correlation between an excess of barbiturates, nonbarbiturate hypnotics, and other psychotropic drugs and an increased risk of falling. This effect is related to the elimination half-life of the drug. In one study, persons treated with hypnotic-anxiolytics (having a half-life of <24 hours) had no increased risk of hip fractures, whereas longer-acting drugs such as tricyclic antidepressants and antipsychotics increased the relative risk by 1.8 and 2.0, respectively. The increased falls were attributed both to the drugs' sedative activity and to the α-adrenergic blockade, which increases the likelihood of orthostatic hypotension. The risk is associated with current usage only.

Drugs that influence bone remodeling, and hence bone mass, need to be documented and quantified, and their continued use reassessed. For example, both exogenous thyroid (in a dose equivalent to 3 grains of the natural extract) and the commonly used diuretic furosemide are associated with a measurable and excessive urinary calcium loss. Thiazide diuretics have calcium-retaining properties, and their long-term use is associated with a lessened risk of hip fracture.

Appropriate calcium and vitamin D nutriture is fundamental to normal bone health. This is especially true in the elderly, who:

- May be less able to afford calcium-rich foods
- Have a tendency to lactose intolerance
- Are less exposed to sunshine.

The consumption of aluminum-containing antacids and/or gastrointestinal complaints associated with impaired calcium absorption need to be considered. Methods of evaluating a patient's calcium intake utilizing tables that list calcium-containing foods and their calcium content are readily available, and are easily calculated by the patient (see Chapter 10, *Calcium, Vitamin D, Vitamin A, Vitamin C, and Vitamin K*). This serves as an educational exercise as well. Calcium-intake guidelines include the following:

- A minimum calcium intake of 1500 mg/day should be the goal, and deficits in the diet should be remedied by appropriate calcium and vitamin D supplements.

- Calcium supplementation in women with low calcium intake can prevent further bone loss.
- Women with established osteoporosis often overcompensate. They should be reminded that an excess intake of calcium (>2000 mg/day) can actually inhibit the bone remodeling cycle, while vitamin D intake should be kept at <1000 IU/day. Values in excess of this amount can mobilize bone mineral and increase the daily calcium loss.

Regular weight-bearing exercise is a stimulant of bone remodeling. The type and amount of exercise need to be carefully evaluated both for efficacy and safety. Apart from the obvious concern of potential fracture, the prescribed exercise should not be injurious to joints and ligaments.

Finally, lifestyle factors such as alcohol and caffeine consumption, as well as cigarette smoking, need to be evaluated because all can contribute significantly to bone loss.

■ Body Composition and Frame

Recent studies have shown that bone mass may not be closely related to many "predisposing" historical factors typically associated with osteoporosis but that the patient's body composition, skeletal frame size, and muscle mass may be helpful. These can be readily assessed by an assistant without the need for specialized equipment.

The body mass index (BMI)—which reflects the percentage of body fat—is determined by the formula: weight in kilograms/height in meters squared:

$$\text{BMI} = \frac{\text{weight (kg)}}{\text{height (m}^2)}$$

For convenience, tables are available that allow for the conversion of pounds and inches as well. Values >27.3 kg/m² in women are indicative of obesity (Tables 8.1 and 8.2). An alternative, but more time-consuming approach, is to measure skinfold thickness at the:

- Triceps
- Suprailiac
- Midthigh.

Osteoporosis is less frequent in obese women.

Women with small frames generally have less bone mass and a greater tendency to develop osteoporosis. Skeletal frame can be estimated by measuring the patient's elbow width. Extend the patient's arm and bend the forearm upward at a 90° angle. With calipers, measure the distance between the medial and lateral condyles of the elbow and compare with the measurements noted in Table 8.3.

Muscle mass can be gauged by measuring the cross-section of the midupper arm circumference in centimeters and the triceps skinfold thickness in millimeters. Using an available nomogram, the upper arm muscle circumference can be established. This is well accepted as a sensitive index of body protein reserves and, by inference, muscle strength. Studies have shown a direct correlation between upper arm muscle strength and lumbar and femoral neck bone mass.

None of the above techniques have been validated in prospective studies, but clinical decisions can be consolidated by combining body composition analysis with bone mass measurement of the appendicular or axial skeleton. More precise body composition studies are possible with total body analysis using dual-energy radiography.

■ The Skeleton

Loss of height is usually the patient's first intimation of developing osteoporosis. Height is only lost in

TABLE 8.1 — ASSESSING IDEAL BODY WEIGHT

| Height* | Ideal Weight* Ranges for Women by Frame Size | | | | | | Suggested Weights* for Adults† | |
| | Metropolitan Life, 1959 | | | Metropolitan Life, 1983 | | | USDA, 1990 | |
	Small	Medium	Large	Small	Medium	Large	19-34 years old	≥ 35 years old
5' 0"	98-106	103-115	111-127	103-115	112-126	122-137	97-128	108-138
5' 1"	101-109	106-118	114-130	105-118	115-129	125-140	101-132	111-143
5' 2"	104-112	109-122	117-134	108-121	118-132	128-144	104-137	115-148
5' 3"	107-115	112-126	121-138	111-124	121-135	131-148	107-141	119-152
5' 4"	110-119	116-131	125-142	114-127	124-138	134-152	111-146	122-157
5' 5"	114-123	120-135	129-146	117-130	127-141	137-156	114-150	126-162
5' 6"	118-127	124-139	133-150	120-133	130-144	140-160	118-155	130-167
5' 7"	122-131	128-143	137-154	123-136	133-147	143-164	121-160	134-172
5' 8"	126-136	132-147	141-159	126-139	136-150	146-167	125-164	138-178
5' 9"	130-140	136-151	145-164	129-142	139-153	149-170	129-169	142-183
5' 10"	134-144	140-155	149-169	132-145	142-156	152-173	132-174	146-188

* All height figures are without shoes; all weight figures are without clothing.

† The USDA table makes no distinction between suggested weights for men and women, noting only that "the higher weights in the ranges generally apply to men, who tend to have more muscle and bone; the lower weights more often apply to women, who have less muscle and bone."

8

TABLE 8.2 — BODY COMPOSITION: DETERMINING BODY MASS INDEX

Find present weight in the left-hand column and read across to the column with height.
A body mass index of 27.3 means individual is moderately overweight; one of 32.3 indicates severe obesity.

Weight (lb)	Height (inches)																
	58	59	60	61	62	63	64	65	66	67	68	69	70	71	72	73	74
110	23.0	22.2	21.5	20.8	20.1	19.5	18.9	18.3	17.8	17.2	16.7	16.2	15.8	15.3	14.9	14.5	14.1
115	24.0	23.2	22.5	21.7	21.0	20.4	19.7	19.1	18.6	18.0	17.5	17.0	16.5	16.0	15.6	15.2	14.8
120	25.1	24.2	23.4	22.7	21.9	21.3	20.6	20.0	19.4	18.8	18.2	17.7	17.2	16.7	16.3	15.8	15.4
125	26.1	25.2	24.4	23.6	22.9	22.1	21.5	20.8	20.2	19.6	19.0	18.5	17.9	17.4	17.0	16.5	16.0
130	27.2	26.3	25.4	24.6	23.8	23.0	22.3	21.6	21.0	20.4	19.8	19.2	18.7	18.1	17.6	17.2	16.7
135	28.2	27.3	26.4	25.5	24.7	23.9	23.2	22.5	21.8	21.1	20.5	19.9	19.4	18.8	18.3	17.8	17.3
140	29.3	28.3	27.3	26.5	25.6	24.8	24.0	23.3	22.6	21.9	21.3	20.7	20.1	19.5	19.0	18.5	18.0
145	30.3	29.3	28.3	27.4	26.5	25.7	24.9	24.1	23.4	22.7	22.0	21.4	20.8	20.2	19.7	19.1	18.6
150	31.4	30.3	29.3	28.3	27.4	26.6	25.7	25.0	24.2	23.5	22.8	22.2	21.5	20.9	20.3	19.8	19.3
155	32.4	31.5	30.5	29.3	28.4	27.5	26.6	25.8	25.0	24.3	23.6	22.9	22.2	21.6	21.0	20.4	19.9
160	33.4	32.3	31.2	30.2	29.3	28.3	27.5	26.6	25.8	25.1	24.3	23.6	23.0	22.3	21.7	21.1	20.5
165	34.5	33.3	32.2	31.2	30.2	29.2	28.3	27.5	26.6	25.8	25.1	24.4	23.7	23.0	22.4	21.8	21.2

170	21.8	22.4	23.1	23.7	24.4	25.1	25.8	26.6	27.4	28.3	29.2	30.1	31.1	32.1	33.2	34.3	35.5
175	22.5	23.1	23.7	24.4	25.1	25.8	26.6	27.4	28.2	29.1	30.0	31.0	32.0	33.1	34.2	35.3	36.6
180	23.1	23.7	24.4	25.1	25.8	26.6	27.4	28.2	29.1	30.0	30.9	31.9	32.9	34.0	35.2	36.4	37.6
185	23.8	24.4	25.1	25.8	26.5	27.3	28.1	29.0	29.9	30.8	31.8	32.8	33.8	35.0	36.1	37.4	38.7
190	24.4	25.1	25.8	26.5	27.3	28.1	28.9	29.8	30.7	31.6	32.6	33.7	34.8	35.9	37.1	38.4	39.7
195	25.0	25.7	26.4	27.2	28.0	28.8	29.6	30.5	31.5	32.4	33.5	34.5	35.7	36.8	38.1	39.4	40.8
200	25.7	26.4	27.1	27.9	28.7	29.5	30.4	31.3	32.3	33.3	34.3	35.4	36.6	37.8	39.1	40.4	41.8
205	26.3	27.0	27.8	28.6	29.4	30.3	31.2	32.1	33.1	34.1	35.2	36.3	37.5	38.7	40.0	41.4	42.8
210	27.0	27.7	28.5	29.3	30.1	31.0	31.9	32.9	33.9	34.9	36.0	37.2	38.4	39.7	41.0	42.4	43.9
215	27.6	28.4	29.2	30.0	30.8	31.8	32.7	33.7	34.7	35.8	36.9	38.1	39.3	40.6	42.0	43.4	44.9
220	28.2	29.0	29.8	30.7	31.6	32.5	33.5	34.5	35.5	36.6	37.8	39.0	40.2	41.6	43.0	44.4	46.0
225	28.9	29.7	30.5	31.4	32.3	33.2	34.2	35.2	36.3	37.4	28.6	39.9	41.2	42.5	43.9	45.4	47.0
230	29.5	30.3	31.2	32.1	33.0	34.0	35.0	36.0	37.1	38.3	39.5	40.7	42.1	43.5	44.9	46.5	48.1
235	30.2	31.0	31.9	32.8	33.7	34.7	35.7	36.8	37.9	39.1	40.3	41.6	43.0	44.4	45.9	47.5	49.1
240	30.8	31.7	32.6	33.5	34.4	35.4	36.5	37.6	38.7	39.9	41.2	42.5	43.9	45.3	46.9	48.5	50.2
245	31.5	32.3	33.2	34.2	35.2	36.2	37.3	38.4	39.5	40.8	42.1	43.4	44.8	46.3	47.8	49.5	51.2
250	32.1	33.0	33.9	34.9	35.9	36.9	38.0	39.2	40.4	41.6	42.9	44.3	45.7	47.2	48.8	50.5	52.3

8

TABLE 8.3 — DETERMINING SKELETAL FRAME SIZE

Measure elbow breadth using the instructions as described in this section under *Body Composition and Frame*. Compare measurement with those in the tables here. These tables list the elbow measurements for women of medium frame at various heights. Measurements lower than those listed indicate a small frame, while higher measurements indicate a large frame.

Height (in 1-in heels)	Elbow Breadth (in)
4' 10" – 4' 11"	$2^{1}/_{4} - 2^{1}/_{2}$
5' 0" – 5' 3"	$2^{1}/_{4} - 2^{1}/_{2}$
5' 4" – 5' 7"	$2^{3}/_{8} - 2^{5}/_{8}$
5' 8" – 5' 11"	$2^{3}/_{8} - 2^{5}/_{8}$
6' 0"	$2^{1}/_{2} - 2^{3}/_{4}$

the vertebral column; the hip-to-heel length remains constant. A more accurate clinical assessment of vertebral height loss is obtained by assessing the crown-to-rump height with the patient seated on a firm stool. A tape measure should be positioned on the wall behind the stool with the zero mark at the seat level (Figure 8.1).

The patient's posture and shape of the spine provide valuable clinical clues, especially when evaluating back pain. Dorsal kyphosis, scoliosis, the presence/absence of appropriate lumbar lordosis, shoulder height, leg length disparity, and pelvic tilt or rotation are all important clinical signs. Figures 8.2 and 8.3 illustrate how to assess some of these features as well as useful bony landmarks.

■ Muscle Strength

Much of the pain experienced by patients with established osteoporosis is muscular in origin. For ex-

FIGURE 8.1 — CROWN-TO-RUMP HEIGHT

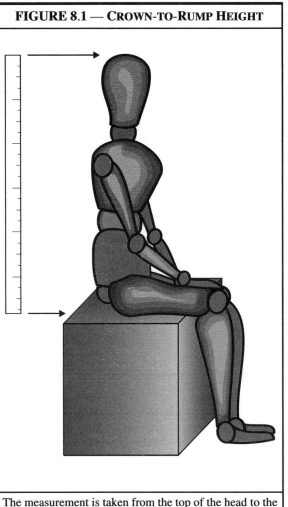

The measurement is taken from the top of the head to the bottom of the spine while the patient is seated on a stool. When crown-to-rump measurements are compared over a number of years, they can help assess whether more than the average loss of stature that occurs with normal aging (a possible sign of vertebral fractures and osteoporosis) is occurring.

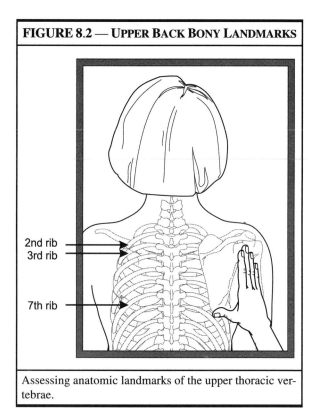

FIGURE 8.2 — UPPER BACK BONY LANDMARKS

2nd rib
3rd rib

7th rib

Assessing anatomic landmarks of the upper thoracic vertebrae.

ample, the typical "burning" pain situated in the mid-thoracic region lateral to the spine is due to excess stress placed on the rhomboid muscles from the compensatory forward rotation of the scapula. The rhomboid major and minor originate from C7 and T4, and extend obliquely downward and laterally to insert into the medial border of the scapula (Figure 8.4). Adopting a military position of "attention," with the shoulders back, relieves this pain. This is a useful confirmatory clinical sign.

Another frequent site of pain is the lower back just above the posterior superior iliac crest. This is frequently associated with lumbar scoliosis and para-

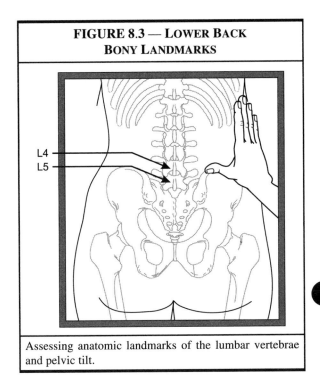

FIGURE 8.3 — LOWER BACK BONY LANDMARKS

L4

L5

Assessing anatomic landmarks of the lumbar vertebrae and pelvic tilt.

vertebral muscle spasm (Figure 8.5). The latter often has the feel of a tense cord and is easily distinguished from the contralateral paravertebral muscle mass.

Disparity in the leg length and/or pelvic rotation produces a "shearing" effect on one sacroiliac joint with "compression" on the other, resulting in lumbosacral strain and pain (Figure 8.6), symptoms that may be aggravated by weakness of the muscular stabilizers of the area: the abdominals, gluteus maximus, and hamstring muscles.

Assessment of muscle spasm, tenderness, and strength helps determine both the cause of the patient's discomfort and the need for specific treatment, such as physical therapy. Figures 8.7, 8.8, 8.9, and 8.10 illustrate simple methods for testing relevant lower body

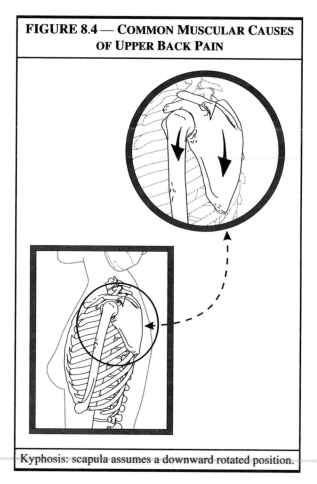

FIGURE 8.4 — COMMON MUSCULAR CAUSES OF UPPER BACK PAIN

Kyphosis: scapula assumes a downward rotated position.

muscle strength: iliopsoas (hip flexor); gluteus maximus (hip extensor); gluteus minimus (hip abduction); and, the adductor group on the medial aspect of the thigh. Strong muscles, including the abdominal and back extensor muscle group, provide more support of joints and an enhanced stability, with a lessened chance of falling.

C7

T5

- - - - - Normal position of scapula

Rhomboid muscle spasm due to forward rotation of scapula.

■ Balance, Falls, and Fractures

More than 25% of persons over 65 years of age fall annually; 5% of these falls will result in a fracture. Falls may be due to neurologic problems, orthostatic hypotension, or a decline in musculoskeletal function.

In screening for a tendency to fall, women should be asked whether they experience dizziness. If so, it is helpful to differentiate among vertigo, syncope, and light-headedness (Table 8.4). Vertigo is associated with a sense of rotation of either the patient or the environment, and is almost always associated with nystagmus,

FIGURE 8.5 — PARAVERTEBRAL MUSCLE SPASM

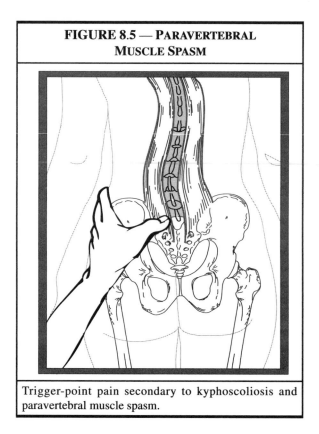

Trigger-point pain secondary to kyphoscoliosis and paravertebral muscle spasm.

poor balance, and autonomic symptoms. Vestibular dysfunction is usually the primary problem. Syncope is defined as a brief loss of consciousness due to cerebral ischemia, vasovagal attacks, orthostatic hypotension, carotid sinus syncope, and cardiac abnormalities, all of which need to be evaluated. Light-headedness describes symptoms of dizziness without nystagmus or loss of consciousness and involves diverse conditions such as hypoglycemia, hypothyroidism, hyperventilation, visual malfunction, and disequilibrium.

To test for orthostatic hypotension, the blood pressure should be taken in a supine or sitting position,

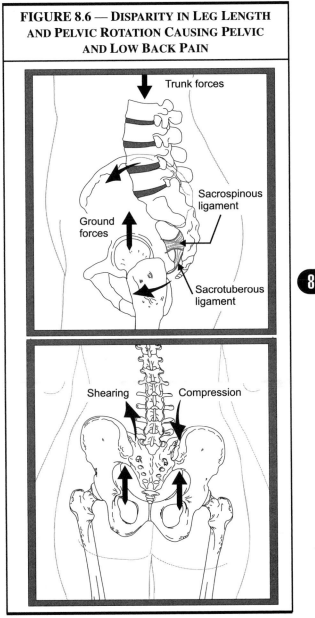

FIGURE 8.6 — DISPARITY IN LEG LENGTH AND PELVIC ROTATION CAUSING PELVIC AND LOW BACK PAIN

Trunk forces

Ground forces

Sacrospinous ligament

Sacrotuberous ligament

Shearing

Compression

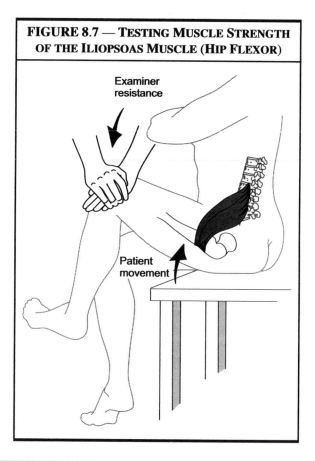

FIGURE 8.7 — TESTING MUSCLE STRENGTH OF THE ILIOPSOAS MUSCLE (HIP FLEXOR)

Examiner resistance

Patient movement

and then with the patient standing. The patient's blood pressure should be measured within 30 seconds of standing and again 3 minutes later. A drop in systolic blood pressure of 20 mm Hg and 10 mm Hg in diastolic pressure is indicative of postural hypotension. If the pulse rate does not increase, a primary autonomic disturbance is the probable cause of the hypotension.

Other tests include:

- Observation for nystagmus, spontaneous and induced

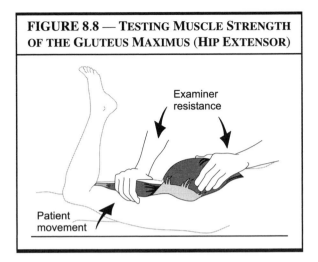

FIGURE 8.8 — TESTING MUSCLE STRENGTH OF THE GLUTEUS MAXIMUS (HIP EXTENSOR)

Examiner resistance

Patient movement

- Romberg's maneuver, with eyes closed and open
- Finger-to-nose test with eyes closed
- Standing on one leg
- Standing on one leg with the heel of the other on the contralateral knee
- Walking on a straight line with eyes looking forward
- One foot placed in front of the other.

Disparity in leg length is associated with both hip and low back pain and may cause imbalance. Measurements are usually taken from the anterior superior iliac crest to the medial malleolus (Figure 8.11-A). Figures 8.11-B and 8.11-C also illustrate how observation of flexed knees placed side by side with the patient supine can differentiate between leg-length disparity due to the femur or lower leg.

The osteoporosis clinical-examination form used at the Women's Medical and Diagnostic Center, Gainesville, Florida, is shown in Figure 8.12.

FIGURE 8.9 — TESTING MUSCLE STRENGTH OF HIP ABDUCTORS: GLUTEUS MINIMUS

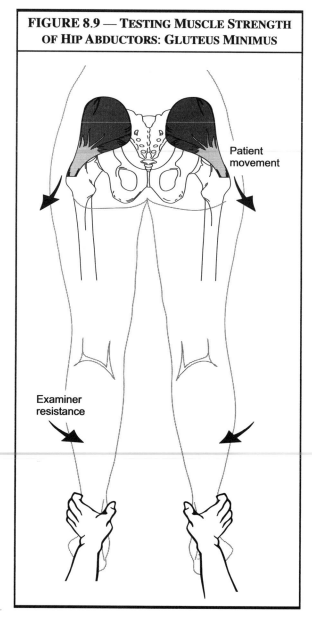

Patient movement

Examiner resistance

FIGURE 8.10 — TESTING MUSCLE STRENGTH OF HIP ABDUCTORS: ADDUCTORS

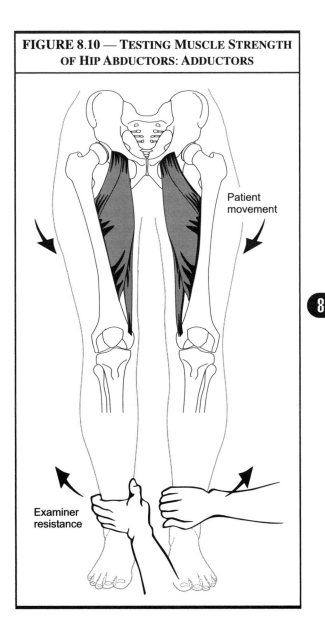

Patient movement

Examiner resistance

TABLE 8.4 — EVALUATION OF DIZZINESS			
	Vertigo	**Syncope**	**Light-Headedness**
Primary symptom	Rotation of patient or environment	Brief loss of consciousness	Dizziness without nystagmus or loss of consciousness
Specific features	Nystagmus Poor balance	Prodromal symptoms Orthostatic hypotension	Hypoglycemia Stress Drugs Hyperventilation
Associated conditions	*Vestibular Apparatus* Benign positional vertigo Ménière's disease Vestibular neuronitis Acoustic neuroma Labyrinthitis	*Cerebral Ischemia* Vasodepressor syncope Orthostatic syncope Carotid sinus syncope Cardiac abnormalities Micturition syncope	*Central Nervous System* Hypoglycemia Hypothyroidism Hyperventilation Visual malfunction Disequilibrium
Primary assessment	Neurologic	Cardiovascular	Metabolic Endocrine Central nervous system

SUGGESTED READING

Bevier WC, Wiswell RA, Pyka G, Kozak KC, Newhall KM, Marcus R. Relationship of body composition, muscle strength, and aerobic capacity to bone mineral density in older men and women. *J Bone Miner Res*. 1989;4:421-432.

Cummings SR, Kelsey JL, Nevitt MC, O'Dowd KJ. Epidemiology of osteoporosis and osteoporotic fractures. *Epidemiol Rev*. 1985; 7:178-208.

Dawson-Hughes B, Dallal GE, Krall EA, Sadowski L, Sahyoun N, Tannenbaum S. A controlled trial of the effect of calcium supplementation on bone density in postmenopausal women. *N Engl J Med*. 1990;323:878-883.

Gryfe CI, Amies A, Ashley MJ. A longitudinal study of falls in an elderly population: I. Incidence and morbidity. *Age Ageing*. 1977; 6:201-210.

Mazess RB, Barden HS, Bisek JP, Hanson J. Dual-energy x-ray absorptiometry for total-body and regional bone-mineral and soft-tissue composition. *Am J Clin Nutr*. 1990;51:1106-1112.

Nevitt MC, Cummings SR, Kidd S, Black D. Risk factors for recurrent nonsyncopal falls. A prospective study. *JAMA*. 1989;261: 2663-2668.

Notelovitz M. The role of the gynecologist in osteoporosis prevention: a clinical approach. *Clin Obstet Gynecol*. 1987;30:871-882.

Ooms ME, Lips P, Van Lingen A, Valkenburg HA. Determinants of bone mineral density and risk factors for osteoporosis in healthy elderly women. *J Bone Miner Res*. 1993;8:669-675.

Pocock N, Eisman J, Gwinn T, et al. Muscle strength, physical fitness, and weight but not age predict femoral neck bone mass. *J Bone Miner Res*. 1989;4:441-448.

Ray WA, Griffin MR, Downey W, Melton LJ III. Long-term use of thiazide diuretics and risk of hip fracture. *Lancet*. 1989;1:687-690.

Ray WA, Griffin MR, Schaffner W, Baugh DK, Melton LJ III. Psychotropic drug use and the risk of hip fracture. *N Engl J Med*. 1987;316:363-369.

Riggs BL, Melton LJ III. Involutional osteoporosis. *N Engl J Med*. 1986;314:1676-1686.

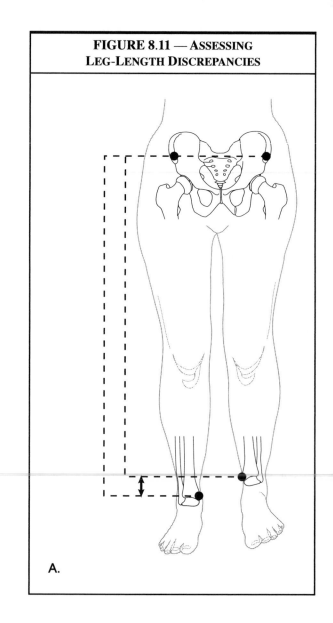

FIGURE 8.11 — ASSESSING LEG-LENGTH DISCREPANCIES

A.

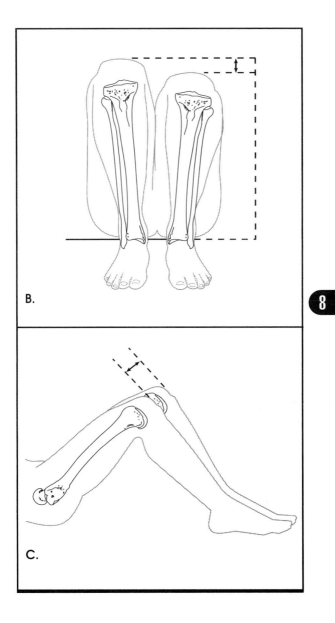

B.

C.

FIGURE 8.12 — PATIENT EXAMINATION FORM

Name: _____

Chart #: _____

Date of Exam: _____

Anthropometrics:

| Max Height _____ | Crown to Rump _____ | Change in Height _____ | Weight _____ | BMI _____ | Change in Weight _____ |

Blood Pressure:

Sitting: _____ Systolic: _____ Diastolic: _____

Standing: _____ Systolic: _____ Diastolic: _____

Positional vertigo: ☐ No ☐ Yes   Latency period: _____

Examination of Back:

PROFILE:

Shoulder height and position: _____

Lumbar curve: _____

Dorsal kyphosis: ☐ No ☐ Yes If YES, site: _____

Scoliosis: ☐ No ☐ Yes If YES, site: _____

	NORMAL	ABNORMAL
	▒▒▒	▒▒▒
	▒▒▒	▒▒▒

PAIN: Present: □No □Yes If YES, site: _____
    Percussion only: _____ Site: _____

MOVEMENT: Flexion: _____ Extension: _____
    Lateral: _____ Rotation: _____

EXTENSOR
MUSCLES: Spasm: _____ □No □Yes If YES, site: _____

OTHER: _____

Balance:

           Spontaneous _____ Induced _____ Positional _____

Nystagmus:

Romberg test:

Finger-nose test:

Heel-shin test:

Line-walk test:

Single-leg balance:

LEG:	LEFT	RIGHT	COMMENT
Length:			
Rotational:			
Flexion:			
Extension:			

Bone Mineral Laboratory Patient Evaluation:

Visit: 1 2 3 4 5 6 7 8 9 10

Name:

Date of Exam: _____

Patient Referral: _____

NLD   WB   SP   FEM

Climacteric History:

Age: _____   LMP: _____   ☐Pre- ☐Peri- ☐Post-menopause

☐Natural ☐Surgical

Years since menopause: _____

Special Features: _____

Systemic Inquiry:

Illness: _____

Fractures: _____

Back pain: _____

Lifestyle:

Exercise: _____

Smoking: _____

Alcohol: _____

Caffeine: Coffee: _____

Tea: _____   Cola: _____

Medications:

Nonprescription: _____

Other: _____

144

Prescription: _____

_____

Hormones: _____

Vitamins/minerals: _____

_____

Height: _____ Weight: _____ BP: _____

Calcium/Vitamin D Assessment::

	Calcium	Vitamin D
Dietary	_____	_____
Supplement	_____	_____
Total intake	_____	_____
OTHER: _____		

Recommendations:

_____
_____
_____
_____
_____
_____
_____
_____
_____
_____

9   Exercise Prescription

The prevention of osteoporosis starts with the onset of the menarche. An individual's ultimate risk of osteoporosis is directly proportional to the amount of bone mineral present prior to the onset of her menopause. A combination of exercise, appropriate nutrition, and a healthy lifestyle maximizes bone mineral accrual and results in optimal peak bone mass (Figure 2.9). Normal ovarian function is also essential to this process. A therapeutic triangle that can be applied to women of any age has been proposed:

- Exercise to stimulate new bone formation
- Good nutrition (calcium and vitamin D) to mineralize the newly formed osteoid
- An estrogen-replete state (endogenous or exogenous) to modulate the rate of bone loss.

Exercise is a known initiator of the bone remodeling cycle because mechanical loading, muscular activity, and gravity stimulate the bone cells to differentiate and grow, modulated by osteocyte activity. As illustrated in Figure 2.7, osteocytes function as both the bone mechanicoreceptors that respond to mechanical strains (exercise) and as modulators of osteoclast activity in bone resorption, and stimulation of osteoblasts and new bone formulations. Osteocytes have both androgen and estrogen receptors and are down-regulated when deprived of estrogen.

Bone mineral maintenance or hypertrophy depends on:

- When exercise is initiated
- The type of exercise
- Frequency of exercise
- Use of gravity during exercise.

Exercise in young girls has at least two positive outcomes: an increase in bone mass and improved bone geometry (a significant increase in the cross-sectional area of the femoral neck and a reduced endosteal expansion). This can be achieved by 2-foot jumps off a 61-cm box three times a week. This generates a ground-reaction force equivalent to eight times body weight.

Bone remodeling responds best to short periods of relatively rapid repetitions and is also site-specific. Female professional tennis players were found to have greater overall bone mass than age-matched casual tennis players and a 28.4% greater cortical thickness in the dominant arm when compared with their own and a control group's nondominant arm. The effect of gravity was also seen in a study of collegiate tennis players and swimmers. Highly trained intercollegiate tennis athletes (weight-bearing) had significantly greater lumbar bone mass evaluated by dual-photon absorptiometry (DPA) when compared with age-matched competitive swimmers (non–weight-bearing).

The positive effect of exercise on bone mass may be related to an increase in the muscle mass. Studies have shown relationships between physical activity, psoas muscle mass, and lumbar vertebrae ash weight in premenopausal women and between spine bone mineral content and back extensor muscle strength in postmenopausal women.

Muscle strength in both biceps and quadriceps is an independent predictor of bone mass in the:
- Proximal femur
- Lumbar spine
- Forearm.

The fact that bicep muscle strength correlates with lumbar bone mineral density (BMD) suggests a systemic effect of exercise. Grip strength correlates significantly with bone density in elderly women (60 to

84 years of age). Loss of hand-grip strength precedes bone mineral loss and is a useful way of identifying the early phase of bone loss. Premenopausal exercise-enhanced BMD is maintained postmenopausally provided the women continue to exercise.

Excessive exercise may be harmful, however. Women marathon runners whose activity is associated with exercise-induced amenorrhea have reduced lumbar BMD with normal or minimally reduced cortical bone. This bone loss has been attributed to a deficiency of estrogen associated with lost body fat. This hypothesis is supported by the finding of an increase in bone mass after estrogen levels in amenorrheic runners returned to normal. Although an estrogen-replete state is probably needed for maximal osteogenic results, the actual cause of exercise-induced osteopenia may be confounded by other factors. For example, high and persistent strains have been found to decrease ERα receptor expression in osteocytes. A more esoteric reason may be zinc deficiency. Zinc is an essential trace element required for bone growth and stimulation of bone formation. A major source of zinc loss is sweat, which increases with excess exercise.

Exercise and Calcium

Exercise is directly associated with the laying down of matrix on the remodeling surface of the trabeculae and cortices of bone. The need for exogenous calcium to meet these increased demands may be a critical factor in maximizing exercise-induced osteogenesis. This may explain why exercising amenorrheic women have lower levels of trabecular, but not cortical, bone mineral when compared with menstruating controls. Although both groups in one study consumed the currently recommended elemental calcium dietary allowance of 800 mg/day, it is clearly established that amenorrheic women actually require 1500 mg/day because of their low-estrogen states (see Chapter 10, *Calcium, Vitamin D, Vitamin A, Vitamin C, and Vitamin K*).

The need for extra calcium in exercising women is supported by a recent cross-sectional study that showed improved bone mineral accretion in women with higher calcium intake and equal energy expenditure. The authors concluded that if their cross-sectional data are confirmed by longitudinal studies, the bone mass accrual from exercise and diet alone could delay the average age of osteoporotic fractures by 10 years.

Exercise and Estrogen

Because exercise stimulates osteogenesis, a recent study evaluated the effect of estrogen therapy plus variable resistance weight training to see if the combined treatment would have an additive effect on bone mineral accrual. Twenty matched surgically menopausal women treated with 0.625 mg/day conjugated equine estrogen were studied; nine of the women also participated in a closely monitored exercise program using Nautilus muscle-strengthening equipment. After 1 year, the exercising group increased bone mineral content of the spine (as measured by total body DPA) by 8.3% ± 5.3% (P <0.01); the estrogen-only group maintained their axial bone mass. A significant increase in the radial midshaft bone density of the exercising group was found by single-photon absorptiometry (SPA); the estrogen-only group had a nonsignificant decrease in midshaft BMD. Similar results have been reported by others. In one study, the exercise-plus-estrogen group had a 2.7% increase in distal BMD; the control group (exercise alone) lost 2.7%.

These results are indirectly supported by a study of aerobic power and bone mass in premenopausal and postmenopausal women. Physical fitness in young menstruating women (mean age, 31 years) results in an improvement in vertebral bone density (183 ± 7 mg/cm^3) when compared with sedentary controls (163 ± 8 mg/cm^3), although no difference was found in physically active postmenopausal women (mean age, 59 years) and their sedentary controls (112 ± 5 vs 111 ± 5 mg/cm^3). These results correlate with studies of exercise-induced amenorrhea and osteopenia in female athletes.

> **Clinical Message**: Exercise can maintain the bone mass of estrogen-deficient menopausal women, but significant increases in BMD require estrogen substitution.

The Exercise Prescription

The current data are too inconsistent and incomplete to be used to develop a generic exercise program. Based on animal experimental data, an increase in bone mass is induced by intermittent strain at or below physiologic peak strain. Therefore, an individual probably does not need extreme physical activity to produce an osteogenic effect; the remodeling process responds best to changes in the distribution of strain. This suggests that exercise should:
- Be diverse and involve different loading situations
- Involve strains imposed as fast rates, which are more effective in inducing new bone formation
- Require relatively few repetitions for the maximal osteogenic effect.

The author's program starts with muscle-strengthening exercises concentrating on the large muscle groups:
- Quadriceps
- Hamstrings

- Abdominal muscles
- Back muscles
- Upper body, including biceps and triceps.

Patients have to be closely supervised and care must be taken to establish each individual's repetition maximum (RM); the maximum weight that can be lifted with one movement = 1 RM. The program should then be developed to allow for a gradual buildup of muscle strength and endurance. We favor:

- Variable-resistance exercise machines (rather than free weights)
- Routines that allow for three sets (separated by 1-minute rest periods) for each muscle group: 12 repetitions at 50% of RM for flexibility; 10 repetitions at 60% of RM for endurance, and 8 repetitions at 70% of RM for strength. Reassess the RM every 3 months. Strength training in calcium-replete postmenopausal women (mean age 60 years) significantly increased the BMD of the hip in a recent 2-year intervention study. The intensity of the exercise must take into account the presence and degree of osteoporosis-prevalent fragility fractures, and a generic caveat: avoid all exercises that flex the spine
- Three sessions per week devoted to muscle-strengthening exercise.

Aerobic exercise is essential for cardiovascular fitness and may have some benefit on bone as well. Although some researchers found a relationship between aerobic exercise and bone formation for women of all ages (20 to 75 years; mean, 45 years), others have shown this to be true only for younger women (25 to 35 years) and not postmenopausal women (55 to 65 years). In the elderly (mean age 70), maximal aerobic capacity does not correlate with bone density.

The duration of aerobic exercise does influence the ability to maintain bone mass. Studies have shown that women who walk ≥7.5 miles a week have higher mean bone density of the whole body, legs, and trunk than women who walk less than 1 mile per week. Also, recently postmenopausal women (less than 6 years postmenopause) who exercise for 30 minutes (at 70% to 85% of maximum heart rate) 3 times a week on a treadmill are able to attenuate the anticipated postmenopausal rate of bone loss; exercising for 45 minutes at the same intensity results in a slight net gain in bone mass.

Any aerobic exercise program (eg, walking on a treadmill, riding a bicycle ergometer, jogging) must be prescribed after assessment of the individual's cardiovascular fitness. Performance of a graded exercise stress test, together with a study of maximal oxygen uptake, allows for the establishment of four parameters necessary for exercise prescription:

- A definitive measure of the person's physical fitness (maximum oxygen consumption)
- Peak heart rate at maximal physical stress measured by electrocardiogram
- Maximum heart rate that allows for an objective level of exercise-intensity prescription
- The total exercise time; this is an indirect method of establishing the muscle strength and endurance of the quadriceps and hamstrings, muscles essential for effective aerobic exercise.

Depending on the patient's initial level of physical fitness, the program is gradually increased upward until heart rate can be maintained at 70% to 80% of the maximal rate for 30 minutes in three to five exercise sessions per week.

Depending on the individual's interests and the availability of exercise equipment, the aerobic content of the exercise program should alternate:

- Walking on a treadmill
- Climbing a stair machine
- Riding a bicycle
- Using a cross-country ski-type apparatus.

This type of program meets the following criteria:
- The exercise is weight-bearing
- The activity is diverse, vigorous, and not overly repetitive
- The program improves cardiovascular fitness
- Because of the program's diversity, boredom is reduced to a minimum—an essential ingredient to ensure long-term compliance.

Will Exercise Prevent Osteoporosis?

The beneficial effect of exercise on osteogenesis is rapidly lost if the intensity and frequency of exercise diminishes and a sedentary lifestyle is resumed. In one study, 6 months of decreased activity in previously exercising women resulted in a reduction in vertebral bone mass from a 6.1% value above preexercise levels to a value of 1.1% above preexercise levels. One of the major problems involving exercise studies is the difficulty of controlling for other influences on the program, eg, dietary habits, drug use, and everyday physical activities other than those designated by the program. Also, comparisons are frequently made between highly trained athletes and nonexercising controls. When recreational athletes are compared with controls, the differences, if present at all, are much less obvious. The site of measurement (the more labile trabecular compartment versus the more stable cortical bone) and the method of bone density testing are added to the numerous variables that must be controlled and considered before a consensus can be reached. Reliance on BMD testing probably underestimates the effect of exercise on bone strength. For example, exercise redistributes bone mineral from the trabecular compartment to the cortex of the femoral neck. Together with other geometric changes, an increase in bending and torsional strength of the bone results.

Exercise probably does contribute to the prevention and treatment of osteoporosis and should be widely prescribed. An additional benefit of exercise is a lessened risk of falls (especially in the elderly) due to an increase in muscular strength, coordination, and flexibility (Figure 3.3).

SUGGESTED READING

Agre JC. Risk of osteoporosis in women: importance of distinguishing between physical activity and aerobic capacity. *Mayo Clin Proc*. 1993;68:821-822.

Bevier WC, Wiswell RA, Pyka G, Kozak KC, Newhall KM, Marcus R. Relationship of body composition, muscle strength, and aerobic capacity to bone mineral density in older men and women. *J Bone Miner Res*. 1989;4:421-432.

Brewer V, Meyer BM, Keele MS, Upton SJ, Hagan RD. Role of exercise in prevention of involutional bone loss. *Med Sci Sports Exerc*. 1983;15:445-449.

Dalsky GP. Exercise: its effect on bone mineral content. *Clin Obstet Gynecol*. 1987;30:820-832.

Dalsky GP, Stocke KS, Ehsani AA, Slatopolsky E, Lee WC, Birge SJ Jr. Weight-bearing exercise training and lumbar bone mineral content in postmenopausal women. *Ann Intern Med*. 1988;108: 824-828.

Doyle F, Brown J, Lachance C. Relation between bone mass and muscle weight. *Lancet*. 1970;1:391-393.

Drinkwater BL, Nilson K, Chesnut CH III, Bremner WJ, Shainholtz S, Southworth MB. Bone mineral content of amenorrheic and eumenorrheic athletes. *N Engl J Med*. 1984;311:277-281.

Drinkwater BL, Nilson K, Ott S, Chesnut CH III. Bone mineral density after resumption of menses in amenorrheic athletes. *JAMA*. 1986;256:380-382.

Feskanich D, Willett W, Colditz G. Walking and leisure-time activity and risk of hip fracture in postmenopausal women. *JAMA*. 2002;288:2300-2306.

Jacobson PC, Beaver W, Grubb SA, Taft TN, Talmage RV. Bone density in women: college athletes and older athletic women. *J Orthop Res*. 1984;2:328-332.

Jarvinen TL, Kannus P, Sievanen H. Have the DXA-based exercise studies seriously underestimated the effects of mechanical loading on bone? *J Bone Miner Res*. 1999;14:1634-1635.

Kanders B, Dempster DW, Lindsay R. Interaction of calcium nutrition and physical activity on bone mass in young women. *J Bone Miner Res*. 1988;3:145-149.

Kerr D, Ackland T, Maslen B, Morton A, Prince R. Resistance training over 2 years increases bone mass in calcium-replete postmenopausal women. *J Bone Miner Res*. 2001;16:175-181.

Kirk S, Sharp CF, Elbaum N, et al. Effect of long-distance running on bone mass in women. *J Bone Miner Res*. 1989;4:515-522.

Krall EA, Darson-Hughes B. Walking is related to bone density and rates of bone loss. *Am J Med*. 1994;96:20-26.

Kritz-Silverstein D, Barrett-Connor E. Grip strength and bone mineral density in older women. *J Bone Miner Res*. 1994;9:45-51.

Lindberg JS, Powell MR, Hunt MM, Ducey DE, Wade CE. Increased vertebral bone mineral in response to reduced exercise in amenorrheic runners. *West J Med*. 1987;146:39-42.

Linnell SL, Stager JM, Blue PW, Oyster N, Robertshaw D. Bone mineral content and menstrual regularity in female runners. *Med Sci Sports Exerc*. 1984;16:343-348.

Madsen OR, Schaadt O, Bliddal H, Egsmose C, Sylvest J. Relationship between quadriceps strength and bone mineral density of the proximal tibia and distal forearm in women. *J Bone Miner Res*. 1993;8:1439-1444.

Marcus R, Drinkwater B, Dalsky G, et al. Osteoporosis and exercise in women. *Med Sci Sports Exerc*. 1992;24(suppl 6):S301-S307.

Martin D, Notelovitz M. Effects of aerobic training on bone mineral density of postmenopausal women. *J Bone Miner Res*. 1993;8:931-936.

Melton LJ III, Chao EY, Lane J. Biomechanical aspects of fractures. In: Riggs BL, Melton LJ III, eds. *Osteoporosis: Etiology, Diagnosis and Management*. New York, NY: Raven Press; 1988: 111-121.

Nelson ME, Fisher EC, Dilmanian FA, Dallal GE, Evans WJ. A 1-y walking program and increased dietary calcium in postmenopausal women: effects on bone. *Am J Clin Nutr*. 1991;53:1304-1311.

Nilsson BE, Westlin NE. Bone density in athletes. *Clin Orthop*. 1971;77:179-182.

Notelovitz M. Postmenopausal osteoporosis. A practical approach to its prevention. *Acta Obstet Gynecol Scand*. 1986;134(suppl):67-80.

Notelovitz M, Fields C, Caramelli K, Dougherty M, Schwartz AL. Cardiorespiratory fitness evaluation in climacteric women: comparison of two methods. *Am J Obstet Gynecol*. 1986;154:1009-1013.

Notelovitz M, Martin D, Tesar R, et al. Estrogen therapy and variable-resistance weight training increase bone mineral in surgically menopausal women. *J Bone Miner Res*. 1991;6:583-590.

Pocock N, Eisman J, Gwinn T, et al. Muscle strength, physical fitness, and weight but not age predict femoral neck bone mass. *J Bone Miner Res*. 1989;4:441-448.

Prince RL, Smith M, Dick IM, et al. Prevention of postmenopausal osteoporosis. A comparative study of exercise, calcium supplementation, and hormone-replacement therapy. *N Engl J Med*. 1991;325: 1189-1195.

Rigotti NA, Nussbaum SR, Herzog DB, Neer RM. Osteoporosis in women with anorexia nervosa. *N Engl J Med*. 1984;311:1601-1606.

Seco C, Revilla M, Hernandez ER, et al. Effects of zinc supplementation on vertebral and femoral bone mass in rats on strenuous treadmill training exercise. *J Bone Miner Res*. 1998;13:508-512.

Seeman E. An exercise in geometry. *J Bone Miner Res*. 2002;17:373-380. Editorial.

Sinaki M, McPhee MC, Hodgson SF, Merritt JM, Offord KP. Relationship between bone mineral density of spine and strength of back extensors in healthy postmenopausal women. *Mayo Clin Proc*. 1986;61:116-122.

Welten DC, Kemper HC, Post GB, et al. Weight-bearing activity during youth is a more important factor for peak bone mass than calcium intake. *J Bone Miner Res*. 1994;9:1089-1096.

Prior JC, Barr SI, Chow R, Faulkner RA. Prevention and management of osteoporosis: consensus statements from the Scientific Advisory Board of the Osteoporosis Society of Canada. 5. Physical activity as therapy for osteoporosis. *CMAJ*. 1996;155:940-944.

10 Calcium, Vitamin D, Vitamin K, Vitamin C, and Vitamin A

Calcium

The protein matrix of bone consists primarily of collagen embedded in a mucopolysaccharide ground substance and accounts for 35% of the volume of the intercellular material. Bone mineral accounts for the remainder. Hydroxyapatite crystals in the mineralized bone contain significant amounts of sodium, magnesium, carbonate, and citrate ions, but calcium and phosphorus are the principal constituents. Factors that regulate their supply, absorption, deposition, and withdrawal from bone determine bone health.

In the United States, the recommended daily allowances (US-RDA) of calcium for females are as follows:

- Age 1 to 10 (children): 1000 mg/day
- Age 11 to 18 (adolescents): 1600 mg/day
- Age 18 to 50 (adults): 1100 mg/day
- Postmenopausal: 1500 mg/day.

Several investigators have shown that the old US-RDA values allow for certain physiologic needs but are well below the amount of calcium needed to maintain positive bone balance. Heaney and associates found that premenopausal women need 1000 mg/day and postmenopausal women need 1400 mg/day to be in calcium balance.

Two studies have shown that children who took calcium supplements increased their bone mass compared with an unsupplemented peer group, and that

159

bone gain continues up to the age of 30, with the calcium-to-protein ratio of the diet the most important determinant of this gain. Furthermore, both the bone mineral content and mean bone area in calcium-supplemented peripubertal girls (compared with a nonsupplemented peer group) is maintained 3 to 5 years after discontinuation of calcium supplementation.

The higher calcium requirement for postmenopausal women is due to a combination of less efficient calcium absorption from the gut and poorer calcium reabsorption by the kidneys. Treatment of postmenopausal women with estrogen results in better absorption and retention and lowers the daily requirement to 1200 mg/day. The deficiency of calcium in real terms among the majority of postmenopausal white women is actually greater. The average intake of calcium by women between the ages of 40 and 65 varies from 450 to 650 mg/day. Thus the average daily calcium intake for these women should generally be increased by 100% (Figure 10.1).

To estimate a patient's calcium intake, see Table 10.1 and Figure 10.2, which list the calcium content of some common foods and summarize the method of calculating the average daily calcium intake.

■ Calcium Absorption and Supplementation

Facts about calcium absorption include:

- Calcium is absorbed primarily in the small intestine, maximally in the duodenum and proximal jejunum.
- Absorption of calcium is complete within 4 hours of its intake and is more efficient with low amounts of calcium.
- Although 75% of ingested calcium may be absorbed by children during periods of rapid skeletal growth and remodeling, the value decreases to 30% to 50% in adults.

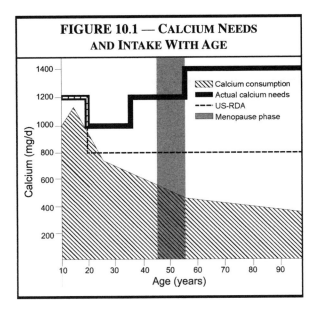

FIGURE 10.1 — CALCIUM NEEDS AND INTAKE WITH AGE

- Intestinal calcium absorption decreases even more in elderly women (>70 years), and especially in women with osteoporosis.
- Despite contrary opinions, calcium is absorbed as efficiently from calcium supplements as from food sources known to be rich in calcium (eg, dairy products). In carefully performed calcium balance studies, researchers were able to establish that it was the amount of available calcium and not the source (milk vs calcium gluconate) that determines whether an individual achieves calcium balance.
- Calcium is needed consistently on a daily basis. Individuals must be given the option of achieving their prescribed amounts by whatever means are convenient, acceptable, and affordable.

Much has been written about the preferred or best type of calcium supplement. The fewer the tablets (and

TABLE 10.1 — CALCIUM (CA) CONTENT OF SOME COMMON FOODS

Food	Amount	Ca (mg)
DAIRY PRODUCTS		
Milk		
Whole (3.5%)	1 cup	288
Nonfat (skim)	1 cup	296
Butter, stick	½ cup	23
Buttermilk	1 cup	296
Cheese		
Blue or Roquefort	1 cu in	54
Camembert	1 wedge	40
Cheddar	1 cu in	129
Cottage	12 oz	320
Parmesan, grated	1 Tbsp	68
Swiss (natural)	1 cu in	139
Swiss (processed)	1 cu in	159
American	1 cu in	122
Cream		
Half-and-Half	1 Tbsp	16
Light	1 Tbsp	15
Sour	1 Tbsp	12
Custard, baked	1 cup	297
Ice cream	1 cup	194
Ice milk		
Hardened	1 cup	204
Soft-serve	1 cup	273
Margarine, stick	½ cup	23
Pudding		
Chocolate	1 cup	250
Vanilla	1 cup	298
Yogurt		
from whole milk	1 cup	272
from partially skimmed	1 cup	294

Food	Amount	Ca (mg)
MEAT, POULTRY & SEAFOOD		
Beef, lean only	2½ oz	10
Chicken breast, fried	2½ oz	9
Eggs		
Whole	1 egg	27
Yolk of egg	1 yolk	24
Scrambled with milk		
and fat	1 egg	51
Clams	3 oz	53
Crabmeat, canned	3 oz	38
Haddock, breaded, fried	3 oz	34
Oysters, raw	1 cup	226
Salmon, pink, canned	3 oz	167
Sardines, canned in		
oil, drained	3 oz	372
Shrimp, canned	3 oz	98
Soups – canned (prepared		
with water)		
Clam chowder	1 cup	34
Cream of chicken	1 cup	24
Cream of mushroom	1 cup	41
Minestrone	1 cup	37
Tuna, canned in oil, drained	3 oz	7
VEGETABLES		
Asparagus, green	1 cup	37
Beans		
Lima	1 cup	80
Red kidney	1 cup	74
Snap (green or yellow)	1 cup	72
Beets	1 cup	29
Broccoli, cooked	1 stalk	158
Brussel sprouts	1 cup	50
Cabbage		
Raw	1 cup	39
Cooked	1 cup	64
Red, raw, coarsely		
shredded	1 cup	29

10

Continued

Food	Amount	Ca (mg)
Carrots	1 cup	45
Cashew nuts	1 cup	53
Cauliflower, cooked	1 cup	25
Celery, pieces	1 cup	39
Collards, cooked	1 cup	289
Mustard greens, cooked	1 cup	193
Onions		
Raw	1 onion	30
Cooked	1 cup	50
Parsnips, cooked	1 cup	70
Peanuts, roasted	1 cup	107
Peas, green	1 cup	44
Pumpkin, canned	1 cup	57
Sauerkraut, canned	1 cup	85
Spinach	1 cup	200
Squash, cooked	1 cup	55
Sweet potatoes	1 med	52
Tomatoes	1 med	24
Tomato catsup	1 cup	60
Turnips, cooked	1 cup	54
Turnip greens, cooked	1 cup	252
FRUITS AND FRUIT PRODUCTS		
Apricots		
Canned in heavy syrup	1 cup	28
Dried, uncooked	1 cup	100
Avocados	1 med	26
Blackberries, raw	1 cup	46
Blueberries, raw	1 cup	21
Cantaloupes, raw, medium	½ melon	27
Cherries, canned, red	1 cup	37
Dates, pitted	1 cup	105
Grapefruit, pink	½ med	20
Grapefruit juice	1 cup	23
Grape juice (canned or bottled)	1 cup	28
Lime juice	1 cup	22
Oranges	1 med	54

Food	Amount	Ca (mg)
Orange juice	1 cup	26
Papayas, raw	1 cup	36
Peaches, dried	1 cup	77
Pineapple	1 cup	27
Pineapple juice, canned	1 cup	37
Plums, canned	1 cup	36
Prunes, cooked	1 cup	60
Prune juice, bottled	1 cup	36
Raspberries, raw	1 cup	27
Rhubarb, cooked	1 cup	212
Strawberries, raw	1 cup	31
Tangerines	1 med	34
Watermelon	4" wedge	30
GRAIN PRODUCTS		
Barley	1 cup	32
Biscuits, homemade	1 biscuit	34
Bran flakes with raisins	1 cup	28
Bread	1 slice	23
Cakes (from mixes)	1 piece	55
Cupcakes (from mixes)	1 small	43
Cornmeal	1 cup	23
Farina, cooked	1 cup	147
Muffins, enriched white flour	1 muffin	42
Oats	1 cup	44
Oatmeal	1 cup	22
Pancakes		
Wheat flour	1 cake	27
Plain or buttermilk	1 cake	58
Pie		
Butterscotch	4" sec	98
Custard	4" sec	125
Mince	4" sec	38
Pecan	4" sec	55
Pumpkin	4" sec	66
Pizza, cheese	5½" sec	107
Rice, cooked	1 cup	21

Continued

10

Food	Amount	Ca (mg)
Rolls		
Hotdog or hamburger	1 roll	30
Hard	1 roll	24
Spaghetti with meat balls		
Home recipe	1 cup	124
Canned	1 cup	53
Waffles		
Enriched flour	1 waffle	85
From mix	1 waffle	179
SUGARS & SWEETS		
Caramels	1 oz	42
Chocolate, milk, plain	1 oz	65
Fudge, plain	1 oz	22
Molasses, blackstrap	1 Tbsp	137
Sherbet	1 cup	31
Sugar, brown	1 cup	187
NUTS & BEANS		
Almonds	½ cup	160
Pecans	½ cup	42
Tofu (soybean curd)	3½ oz	128
Walnuts	½ cup	50

Adapted from Krause MV, Mahan LK. *Food, Nutrition and Diet Therapy*. Philadelphia, Pa: WB Saunders Co; 1979:828.

the less expensive), the more likely it is that individuals will take supplements. Three essential points need emphasis:

- *First*: Only elemental calcium is available for absorption. Calcium carbonate contains 40% of calcium in elemental form; tribasic calcium phosphate, 39%; calcium citrate, 24%; calcium lactate, 13%; and, calcium gluconate, 9%. In clinical terms, the availability of calcium from these sources does not differ significantly, but some researchers have suggested that calcium citrate is more bioavailable than calcium carbonate.

- *Second*: Generic calcium supplements are not always bioavailable. The disintegration and dissolution times of calcium supplements are critical to calcium absorption and can be tested by placing the tablet in white vinegar. The tablet should dissolve within 30 minutes.
- *Third*: The timing of calcium supplementation can theoretically maximize its absorption. Calcium taken several times a day with meals is less likely to saturate the intestinal absorptive mechanism. Calcium also has a diurnal metabolism; it is stored in bone during the day and released during the night. A further consideration is impaired stomach acid production and its effect on calcium absorption, especially in postmenopausal and elderly women. The fractional absorption of calcium citrate and carbonate are similar in normal subjects, but significantly less calcium carbonate is absorbed by achlorhydric women. This can be corrected by taking calcium carbonate with a meal.

The author's approach to calcium supplementation is as follows:

- Supplements no greater than 500 mg/day are taken at night; if more is needed, a twice daily regimen is prescribed.
- In older patients, calcium citrate is prescribed.
- Calcium carbonate, if preferred, must be taken with a meal.

People with special calcium needs are listed in Table 10.2.

FIGURE 10.2 — CALCIUM (CA) INTAKE ASSESSMENT

Name: _____   Date: _____

INSTRUCTIONS: For each of the following foods you consumed in the last 7 days, estimate the total amount for the week and write it in the amount (AMT) column (ie, ½ cup, 6 oz, 5 Tbsp, etc.)

I. DAIRY PRODUCTS

MILK	Measurement	Mg/Cal	AMT	Calcium Total
Whole	1 cup	288		
Low-fat (2%)	1 cup	352		
Skim or buttermilk	1 cup	296		
Nonfat, dry (powder)	¼ cup	220		
Chocolate	1 cup	278		
Condensed, sweetened	1 cup	802		
Evaporated	1 cup	635		
Lactimilk	1 cup			
CHEESE	**Measurement**	**Mg/Cal**	**AMT**	**Calcium Total**
Swiss	1 oz	262		
Cheddar, provolone	1 oz	213		

Edam	1 oz	207
Monterey Jack	1 oz	200
Mozzarella	1 oz	200
Muenster	1 oz	198
American, gouda	1 oz	198
Brick	1 oz	191
Velveeta (cheese food)	2 Tbsp = 1 oz	162
Romano	1 oz	156
Blue	1 oz	150
Parmesan	1 oz	136
Feta	1 oz	100
Ricotta (skim)	1 oz	84
Ricotta (whole)	1 oz	65
Brie	1 oz	52
Camembert	1 oz	30
Cottage, low-fat	1 cup	204
Cottage, regular	1 cup	131

Continued

10

OTHER	Measurement	Mg/Cal	AMT	Calcium Total
Ice cream (hard pack)	1 cup	194		
Ice cream (soft serve)	1 cup	253		
Ice milk (hard pack)	1 cup	204		
Pudding (instant)	1 cup	374		
Pudding (cooked)	1 cup	265		
Custard (baked)	1 cup	265		
Yogurt (low-fat, plain)	1 cup	297		
Yogurt (low-fat fruited)	1 cup	452		
Yogurt (whole milk)	1 cup	275		
Yogurt (custard style)	1 cup	333		
Yogurt (frozen)	1 cup	220		
II. SEAFOOD				
Clams, canned solid/liquid	1 cup	121		
Mackerel, canned solid/liquid	1 cup	552		
Oyster stew, milk/6 oysters/cup	1 cup	274		
Salmon, sockeye, canned solid/liquid w/bones	1 cup	587		
Sardines, canned, 8/can w/bones	4 medium	69		

III. VEGETABLES & NUTS		
Broccoli (frozen, chopped, cooked)	1 cup	100
Bok choy (chopped, cooked)	1 cup	250
Collards (frozen, chopped, cooked)	1 cup	299
Kale (frozen, chopped, cooked)	1 cup	157
Mustard greens (frozen, chopped, cooked)	1 cup	156
Turnip greens (frozen, chopped, cooked)	1 cup	195
Beans, all varieties (dry, cooked, canned, solid/liquid)	1 cup	80
Almonds (shelled, chopped)	1 cup	304
Pecans (shelled, chopped)	1 cup	86
Peanuts (shelled, chopped)	1 cup	104
Mixed nuts, dry roasted peanuts	1 cup	96
Walnuts, English (shelled, chopped)	1 cup	119
IV. MISCELLANEOUS		
Tofu	1 oz	36
Soybeans (cooked, sprouted)	1 cup	54
Sunflower seeds (hulled)	1 cup	174

Continued

10

Cream soups (w/milk)	1 cup	184
Macaroni & cheese (homemade)	1 cup	362
Milk chocolate candy	1 oz	65
Pizza (frozen w/cheese)	4½" arc	89
Carob flour	1 cup	480
Molasses, blackstrap	1 Tbsp	137

V. CALCIUM FORTIFIED FOODS

Citrus Hill orange juice	1 cup	300
Minute Maid orange juice	1 cup	320
Calci-Milk	1 cup	500

Calculated Calcium Intake

Dietary: _____   Supplemental: _____   Total: _____

For average daily intake ÷ 7: _____   Daily intake: _____

Vitamin D Intake Assessment

	Measurement	IU	AMT	Total
Milk	1 cup	100		
Cereal	1 cup	40		

172

Calculated Vitamin D Intake

Dietary: _____   Supplemental: _____   Total: _____

For average daily intake ÷ 7: _____   Daily intake: _____

A WORD ABOUT GETTING ENOUGH CALCIUM

Life Stage (for females)	Recommended Calcium Intake (mg)
Children (ages 1 to 10)	1000
Adolescents (ages 11 to 18) and pregnant/lactating women over age 20	1600
Premenopause (to age 35 with functioning ovaries)	1100
Perimenopause (age 35 to 50 with functioning ovaries)	1200
Postmenopausal (natural or surgical menopause)	1500 to 2000

10

TABLE 10.2 — PERSONS WITH SPECIAL CALCIUM-INTAKE NEEDS

Persons for Whom the 1980 US-RDA for Calcium May Not Be Adequate
- Perimenopausal women
- Estrogen-deprived women
- Persons with exercise-induced amenorrhea
- Persons with certain dietary or lifestyle factors:
  - High protein intake
  - High fiber intake
  - High sodium intake
  - High caffeine intake
  - Use of aluminum-containing antacids
- Persons convalescing from illness, injury, or major surgery
- Following diet-induced weight loss

Persons Not Receiving Even the 1980 US-RDA for Calcium
- Persons with self-selected low calcium intakes
- Persons with anorexia nervosa
- Persons placed on therapeutic low sodium intakes
- Strict vegetarians (vegans)
- Persons placed on low calcium diets for renal stone disease

Heaney RP. *Annu Rev Nutr.* 1993;13:287-316.

■ Protective Effects of Calcium

Can calcium by itself prevent osteoporosis? Until recently, there were no long-term studies showing a decrease in the incidence of osteoporosis-related fractures after nutritional intervention. However, recent studies have concluded that:

- The age-adjusted risk of hip fracture is inversely associated with dietary calcium, whether considered as milligrams per day or as nutrient density, milligrams per 1000 kcal

- In a 14-year prospective follow-up Yugoslavian study, subjects with a calcium intake >765 mg/day had a 60% lower risk of hip fractures when compared with people in certain villages with higher and lower calcium intakes
- Calcium supplementation in women >65 years of age does decrease the prevalence of osteoporotic fractures.

The protective effect of calcium is probably determined by:
- The age at which adequate calcium intake occurs and the lifetime exposure to this intake through the premenopausal, perimenopausal, and postmenopausal years
- An estrogen-replete state, whether the estrogen is from an endogenous or exogenous source. Note: untreated postmenopausal women still synthesize estrogen; the greater this amount, the less the risk of vertebral and hip fracture.

Cross-sectional studies exploring the relationship between calcium use and bone mass will lead to false conclusions if the information is based on the current intake of calcium. The dietary threshold between calcium intake and bone protection is about 800 mg/day. Clinical trials of calcium supplementation have shown reduced rates of bone loss.

Table 10.3 is a guide to some calcium supplements. Costs vary with location.

■ Side Effects of Calcium Supplementation

The only potential side effect of calcium therapy is the development of renal stones, which rarely occurs in women. Renal stones occur in individuals who lack the enzymes necessary to keep the calcium and urine in solution. They are not caused by excessive calcium intake. Calcium citrate inhibits calcium oxalate

TABLE 10.3 — A GUIDE TO CALCIUM SUPPLEMENTS			
Generic (Trade) Name	Total Calcium per Tablet (mg)	Elemental Calcium (mg)	Number of Tablets to Provide 1000 mg Calcium
Calcium carbonate (Apo-Cal, BioCal, Calcarb 600, Calci-Chew, Calciday 667, Calcilac, Calcite 500, Calcium Carbonate/600, Calcium-600, Calcium-Sandoz Forte, Calglycine, Calsan, Caltrate, Caltrate-300, Caltrate-600, Caltrate Chewable, Chooz, Gencalc 600, Gramcal, Mallamint, Nephro-Calci, Os-Cal, Os-Cal 500, Os-Cal Chewable, Oysco, Oysco 500 Chewable, Oyst-Cal, Oyst-Cal 500 Chewable, Oystercal 500, Rolaids-Calcium Rich, Titralac, Tums, Tums E-X)	625 650 750 835 1250 1500	250 260 300 334 500 600	4 4 4 3 2 2
Calcium citrate (Citracal, Citracal Liquitabs)	950	200	5
Calcium gluconate (Calcium Stanley, Kalcinate)	500 650 1000	45 58 90	22 17 11

Calcium lactate (Calcium-Sandoz Forte, Gramcal)	325 650	42 84	24 12
Calcium phosphate, dibasic	500	115	9
Calcium phosphate, tribasic (Posture)	800 1600	304 608	4 2

Adapted from: "Calcium Supplements" in *The Complete Drug Reference*. Yonkers, NY: Consumer Reports Books; 1991; and Griffith HW. *Complete Guide to Prescription and Nonprescription Drugs*. New York, NY: The Berkley Publishing Group; 2003:877-878.

10

crystallization and should, therefore, be the preparation of choice for women at risk of kidney stone formation. Treatment with hydrochlorothiazide diuretics (25 mg to 50 mg daily) also lessens the risk of renal stone formation. In patients at risk, the 24-hour urinary excretion of calcium should be monitored and kept <300 mg/day; with a high fluid intake, the calcium concentration in urine can be kept at a level incompatible with renal stone formation.

■ Calcium-to-Phosphorus Ratio

Earlier studies suggested that an excess of phosphorus-containing foods had a negative impact on bone mineral accrual. This was thought to be mediated through a promotion of urinary calcium excretion. Although this issue is still unresolved, patients should be advised to aim for a calcium-to-phosphorus ratio of 2:1.

The easiest advice to give is to avoid excess of:
- Red meat
- Cola drinks
- Processed foods with phosphorus additives.

Listed in Table 10.4 are various common foods, along with their calcium-to-phosphorus ratio.

Vitamin D

Elderly patients and women with osteoporosis absorb calcium less efficiently. This is believed to be caused by a deficiency of the activated form of vitamin D, $1,25\text{-}(OH)_2D_3$-calcitriol. Vitamin D plays a major role in the absorption of calcium and the maintenance of calcium balance. Because vitamin D is synthesized in the skin in response to solar irradiation, its significance as a nutrient is frequently underestimated. A reduced dietary intake, especially if associated with intestinal malabsorption of fats, can result in the depletion of vitamin D stores in elderly patients who are not exposed to sunlight (Figure 10.3). To ensure an adequate intake of vitamin D in elderly women, the author prescribes one multivitamin tablet per day to provide 400 IU. Some authorities now believe that older women should receive 800 IU of vitamin D per day. Otherwise healthy postmenopausal women with osteoporosis should be tested for vitamin D deficiency. The prevalence of vitamin D insufficiency (25 (OH)D $\leq$15 mg/mL) is strongly correlated with reduced bone mineral density (BMD) of both the spine and the hip.

Certain varieties of hormone therapy influence vitamin D metabolism in the following ways:

- Exogenous estrogen increases $1,25\text{-}(OH)_2D_3$, in part, by increasing vitamin D–binding protein
- The increase in $1,25\text{-}(OH)_2D_3$ is somewhat offset by medroxyprogesterone acetate
- Long-term use of depot medroxyprogesterone acetate is associated with reduced bone mass.

Subclinical vitamin D depletion may predispose the elderly to hip fractures as a result of accelerated cortical bone loss associated with secondary hyperparathyroidism. Vitamin D deficiency also affects muscle strength and body sway—both of which are risk factors for falls and fractures. Vitamin D–deficient individuals have proximal muscle atrophy with loss of type II muscle fibers. This may be mediated via specific vitamin D receptors in muscle. It takes 6 to 12 months of vitamin D supplementation to recover from vitamin D deficiency. Excessive amounts of vitamin D may be even more harmful and lead to an increase in urinary calcium excretion and a further loss of cortical bone. An interesting hypothesis suggests that $1,25\text{-}(OH)_2D_3$ inhibits the proliferation of megakaryocytes that normally promote collagen synthesis. It is currently recommended that dietary and/or supplemental vitamin D should not exceed 1000 IU/day. Parentheti-

TABLE 10.4 — CALCIUM, PHOSPHORUS, AND CALCIUM-TO-PHOSPHORUS RATIO OF COMMON FOODS

	Ca (mg)	P (mg)	Ratio Ca:P
American cheese, 1 slice	188	208	1:1.1
Apple pie, average slice	9	29	1:2.9
Bacon, cooked, 2 thin slices	1	22	1:22.0
Beans, green, canned, 1 cup	81	50	1:0.6
Beef liver, fried, 1 slice	9	405	1:45.0
Beef noodle soup, canned, 1 cup	7	48	1:6.9
Biscuit mix made with milk, 1 biscuit	19	65	1:3.4
Bologna, 1 slice	1	17	1:17.0
Bran flakes with raisins, 1 cup	28	146	1:5.2
Broccoli (frozen), boiled, 1 cup	100	104	1:1.0
Cauliflower (frozen), boiled, 1 cup	31	68	1:2.2
Cheddar cheese, 1 slice	158	100	1:0.6
Cherry pie, average slice	17	30	1:1.8
Chicken, fried, 1 drumstick	6	89	1:14.8
Chicken chow mein without noodles, homemade, 1 cup	58	293	1:5.1
Chicken noodle soup, canned 1 cup	10	36	1:3.6
Chili con carne with beans, canned, 1 cup	82	321	1:3.9
Chocolate chip cookies, 4 homemade	14	40	1:2.9
Chocolate devil's food cake, without icing, 1 cupcake	24	45	1:1.9
Coffee, instant, 1 cup	4	8	1:1.8
Corn-on-the-cob, cooked, 1 ear	2	69	1:34.5
Cottage cheese, large curd, 1 cup	212	342	1:1.61
Danish pastry (plain), 1 piece	21	46	1:2.2
Egg, fried, 1 large	28	102	1:3.6
Flounder filet, baked with butter	23	344	1:15.0
Frankfurter	4	76	1:19.0
French fries, 10 strips	12	87	1:7.3
Ground beef, cooked 3 oz	10	196	1:19.6
Ham, baked, 3 oz	9	201	1:22.3
Hard roll	24	46	1:1.9

	Ca (mg)	P (mg)	Ratio Ca:P
Ice cream, plain, soft-serve, 1 cup	253	199	1:0.8
Lamb chops, loin, broiled, 6 9-oz chops	24	429	1:17.9
Lettuce, shredded, 1 cup	19	14	1:0.7
Lobster Newburg, 1 cup	218	480	1:2.2
Mashed potatoes, with milk, 1 cup	50	103	1:0.8
Milk, whole, 1 cup	288	227	1:2.8
Minestrone soup, canned, 1 cup	37	59	1:1.6
Oatmeal, cooked, 1 cup	22	137	1:6.2
Orange juice, frozen, 6 oz	19	32	1:1.7
Peanut butter, 1 Tbsp	9	61	1:6.8
Peanuts, roasted, salted	21	114	1:5.4
Peas (frozen), boiled, 1 cup	30	138	1:4.6
Popcorn, with oil and salt	1	19	1:19.0
Pork and beans, canned, 1 cup	138	235	1:1.7
Pork chops, broiled, 8 2-oz chops	28	624	1:22.3
Potato chips, 10 chips	8	28	1:3.5
Pretzels, 10 3-ring pretzels	7	39	1:5.6
Puffed rice cereal	3	14	1:4.7
Pumpkin pie, average slice	58	79	1:1.4
Rice, white, cooked, 1 cup	21	57	1:2.7
Rye bread, 1 slice	19	37	1:1.9
Saltines, 10 crackers	6	26	1:4.3
Sesame seeds, hulled, 1 Tbsp	9	47	1:5.2
Shrimp, French fried, 1 oz	20	54	1:2.7
Spaghetti, homemade, with tomato sauce, meatballs, Parmesan cheese	124	236	1:1.9
Spinach, canned, 1 cup	242	53	1:0.2
T-bone steak, cooked, yield from 1 lb raw	24	490	1:20.4
Tomato, 1 average	24	49	1:2.0
Tomato soup, canned, 1 cup	15	34	1:2.3
Tuna, canned, 1 cup	13	374	1:28.8
Vegetable beef soup, canned, 1 cup	12	49	1:4.1
White bread, enriched, 1 slice	24	27	1:1.1
Winter squash, baked, 1 cup	57	98	1:1.7

Abbreviations: Ca, calcium; P, phosphorus.

10

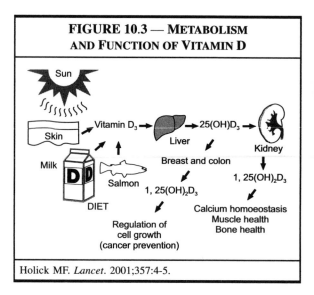

FIGURE 10.3 — METABOLISM AND FUNCTION OF VITAMIN D

Holick MF. *Lancet*. 2001;357:4-5.

cally, the activated form of vitamin D 1,25 $(OH)_2D$ is a potent hormone that regulates cell proliferation and may even limit the metastatic behavior of some cancers.

Vitamin K

Vitamin K is also important for normal bone health; in fact, vitamin K levels are low in hip fracture victims. Vitamin K mediates the gamma carboxylation of glutamic acid residues resulting in:

- Binding of calcium
- Inhibition of mineralization in urine
- Osteoclast chemotaxis
- Synthesis of osteocalcin (bone GLA-protein [BGP]).

Physiologic doses of vitamin K:
- Restore low values of BGP

- Reduce elevated urinary calcium excretion
- Reduce urinary hydroxyproline levels.

There are two sources of vitamin K:
- Vitamin K_1 (phytonadione): This variety is provided by food. The average American diet contains adequate amounts of vitamin K; leafy green vegetables are the best natural source of vitamin K.
- Vitamin K_2 (menaquinone): This form of vitamin K is synthesized by the bacteria in the microflora of the gut. Vitamin K_2 is the main storage form of vitamin K in the liver. A decrease in subclass menaquinone-8 (MK-8) may occur without a decrease in vitamin K_1 and is especially related to an increased risk for hip fracture.

Vitamin C

Vitamin C plays an important role in collagen synthesis and stimulates osteoblast differentiation, including the expression of alkaline phosphatase, a marker of osteoblast formation and function. Vitamin C also modulates osteoclast formation and increases the lifespan of osteoclasts. Although there is no consensus, a recent study involving 994 women concluded that vitamin C supplement use has a beneficial effect on BMD, especially among postmenopausal women who, in addition, are on estrogen therapy and take calcium supplements. The optimal dose of vitamin C is not known, but the highest BMD values are observed in women taking ≥ 1000 mg/day. This association is true for the hip and ultradistal radius, but not the lumbar spine. (Pharmacokinetic studies have shown that the intestinal absorption capacity for ascorbic acid is approximately 3 g/day.)

Vitamin A

In animals, excess amounts of retinoic acid inhibit osteoblast function and stimulate osteoclast formation. This results from the overproduction of cytokines by osteoblasts, which act as messengers to recruit osteoclast precursor cells. Continuous and prolonged stimulation leads to the uncoupling of bone remodeling, progressive bone loss with resulting microarchitectural damage, and fractures. There is also a negative interaction between retinoic acid and 1,25 dihydroxyvitamin D and a reduction in intestinal calcium absorption. The rate of bone loss is fairly rapid. The risk of hip fracture doubles in women consuming >1500 to 2000 µg/day ($\pm$ 4500 IU) of retinol compared with women who consume <500 µg/day.

This relationship is especially true for excess amounts of vitamin A in fortified foods and to a lesser extent for vitamin A supplements. An example, both skim and low-fat milk are fortified with 350 µg/cup; breakfast cereals have 375 µg vitamin A, and margarine (1 tablespoon) about 150 µg vitamin A. Multivitamins contain 1500 µg retinol per tablet. The use of carotene supplements does not increase the risk of hip fractures. Vitamin A is readily absorbed and stored in the body (liver and fat tissue). Vitamin A toxicity may occur from repeated daily doses of 25,000 to 50,000 IU/day (1 IU = 0.3 µg retinol), with the elderly being especially vulnerable. This is because retinol has a longer half-life in the elderly, with higher postprandial serum retinol values and greater amounts of "free" and potentially toxic levels of vitamin A.

Anderson JJ. Oversupplementation of vitamin A and osteoporotic fractures in the elderly: to supplement or not to supplement with vitamin A. *J Bone Miner Res*. 2002;17:1359-1362. Editorial.

Avioli LB. Diseases of bone: calcium, phosphorus and bone metabolism. In: Beeson PB, McDermott W, Wyngaarden JB, eds. *Cecil Textbook of Medicine*. Philadelphia, Pa: WB Saunders Co; 1979:2225-2231.

Bikle DD, Halloran BP, Harris ST, Portale AA. Progestin antagonism of estrogen stimulated 1,25-dihydroxyvitamin D levels. *J Clin Endocrinol Metab*. 1992;75:519-523.

Bonjour JP, Chevalley T, Ammann P, Slosman D, Rizzoli R. Gain in bone mineral mass in prepubertal girls 3-5 years after discontinuation of calcium supplementation: a follow-up study. *Lancet*. 2001;358:1208-1212.

Carr CJ, Shangraw RF. Nutritional and pharmaceutical aspects of calcium supplementation. *Am Pharm*. 1987;NS27:49-57.

Cauley JA, Gutai JP, Kuller LH, et al. Endogenous estrogen levels and calcium intakes in postmenopausal women. Relationships with cortical bone measures. *JAMA*. 1988; 260:3150-3155.

Cundy T, Evans M, Roberts H, Wattie D, Ames R, Reid IR. Bone density in women receiving depot medroxyprogesterone acetate for contraception. *BMJ*. 1991;303:13-16.

Dhesi JK, Bearne LM, Moniz C, et al. Neuromuscular and psychomotor function in elderly subjects who fall and the relationship with vitamin D status. *J Bone Miner Res*. 2002;17:891-897.

Elders PJ, Lips P, Netelenbos JC, et al. Long-term effect of calcium supplementation on bone loss in perimenopausal women. *J Bone Miner Res*. 1994;9:963-970.

Feskanich D, Singh V, Willett WC, Colditz GA. Vitamin A intake and hip fractures among postmenopausal women. *JAMA*. 2002;287:47-54.

Gallagher JC, Riggs BL, DeLuca HF. Effect of estrogen on calcium absorption and serum vitamin D metabolites in postmenopausal osteoporosis. *J Clin Endocrinol Metab*. 1980;51:1359-1364.

10

Gallagher JC, Riggs BL, Eisman J, Hamstra A, Arnaud SB, DeLuca HF. Intestinal calcium absorption and serum vitamin D metabolites in normal subjects and osteoporotic patients: effect of age and dietary calcium. *J Clin Invest*. 1979;64:729-736.

Harvey JA, Zobitz MM, Pak CY. Calcium citrate: reduced propensity for the crystallization of calcium oxalate in urine resulting from induced hypercalciuria of calcium supplementation. *J Clin Endocrinol Metab*. 1985;61:1223-1225.

Heaney RP. Bone mass, nutrition, and other lifestyle factors. *Am J Med*. 1993;95(suppl 5A):29S-33S.

Heaney RP. Nutritional factors in osteoporosis. *Annu Rev Nutr*. 1993;13:287-316.

Heaney RP, Gallagher JC, Johnston CC, Neer R, Parfitt AM, Whedon GD. Calcium nutrition and bone health in the elderly. *Am J Clin Nutr*. 1982;36(suppl 5):986-1013.

Heaney RP, Recker RR, Stegman MR, Moy AJ. Calcium absorption in women: relationships to calcium intake, estrogen status, and age. *J Bone Miner Res*. 1989;4:469-475.

Hodges SJ, Akesson K, Vergnaud P, Obrant K, Delmas PD. Circulating levels of vitamins K_1 and K_2 decreased in elderly women with hip fracture. *J Bone Miner Res*. 1993;8:1241-1245.

Hodges SJ, Pilkington MJ, Stamp TC, et al. Depressed levels of circulating menaquinones in patients with osteoporotic fractures of the spine and femoral neck. *Bone*. 1991;12:387-389.

Holbrook TL, Barrett-Connor E, Wingard DL. Dietary calcium and risk of hip fracture: 14-year prospective population study. *Lancet*. 1988;2:1046-1049.

Holick MF. Sunlight "D"ilemma: risk of skin cancer or bone disease and muscle weakness. *Lancet*. 2001;357:4-6.

Jensen LB, Kollerup G, Quaade F, Sorensen OH. Bone mineral changes in obese women during a moderate weight loss with and without calcium supplementation. *J Bone Miner Res*. 2001;16:141-147.

Johnston CC Jr, Miller JZ, Slemenda CW, et al. Calcium supplementation and increases in bone mineral density in children. *N Engl J Med*. 1992;327:82-87.

Krause MV, Mahan LK. *Food, Nutrition and Diet Therapy*. Philadelphia, Pa: WB Saunders Co; 1979:828.

Lloyd T, Andon MB, Rollings N, et al. Calcium supplementation and bone mineral density in adolescent girls. *JAMA*. 1993;270:841-844.

Matkovic V, Kostial K, Simonovic I, Buzina R, Brodarec A, Nordin BE. Bone status and fracture rates in two regions of Yugoslavia. *Am J Clin Nutr*. 1979;32:540-549.

McCarthy DM, Hibbin JA, Goldman JM. A role for 1,25-dihydroxyvitamin D_3 in control of bone-marrow collagen deposition? *Lancet*. 1984;1:78-80.

Mezquita-Raya P, Munoz-Torres M, Luna JD, et al. Relation between vitamin D insufficiency, bone density, and bone metabolism in healthy postmenopusal women. *J Bone Miner Res*. 2001;16:1408-1415.

Morton DJ, Barrett-Connor EL, Schneider DL. Vitamin C supplement use and bone mineral density in postmenopausal women. *J Bone Miner Res*. 2001;16:135-140.

Murray TM. Prevention and management of osteoporosis: consensus statements from the Scientific Advisory Board of the Osteoporosis Society of Canada. 4. Calcium, nutrition and osteoporosis. *CMAJ*. 1996;155:935-939.

Nicar MJ, Pak CY. Calcium bioavailability from calcium carbonate and calcium citrate. *J Clin Endocrinol Metab*. 1985;61:391-393.

Nordin BE, Horsman A, Crilly RG, Marshall DH, Simpson M. Treatment of spinal osteoporosis in postmenopausal women. *Br Med J*. 1980;280:451-455.

Parfitt AM. Integration of skeletal and mineral homeostasis. In: DeLuca HF, Frost H, Jee W, et al, eds. *Osteoporosis: Recent Advances in Pathogenesis and Treatment*. Baltimore, Md: University Park Press; 1981:115-126.

Recker RR. Calcium absorption and achlorhydria. *N Engl J Med*. 1985;313:70-73.

Recker RR, Davies KM, Hinders SM, Heaney RP, Stegman MR, Kimmel DB. Bone gain in young adult women. *JAMA*. 1992;268: 2403-2408.

Reichel H, Koeffler HP, Norman AW. The role of the vitamin D endocrine system in health and disease. *N Engl J Med*. 1989;320:980-991.

Reid IR, Ames RW, Evans MC, Gamble GD, Sharpe SJ. Effect of calcium supplementation on bone loss in postmenopausal women. *N Engl J Med*. 1993;328:460-464.

Riis B, Thomsen K, Christiansen C. Does calcium supplementation prevent postmenopausal bone loss? A double-blind, controlled clinical study. *N Engl J Med*. 1987;316:173-177.

Sandler RB, Slemenda CW, LaPorte RE, et al. Postmenopausal bone density and milk consumption in childhood and adolescence. *Am J Clin Nutr*. 1985;42:270-274.

Sheikh MS, Santa Ana CA, Nicar MJ, Schiller LR, Fordtran JS. Gastrointestinal absorption of calcium from milk and calcium salts. *N Engl J Med*. 1987;317:532-536.

11   Postmenopausal Hormone Therapy

Estrogen

Based on observational studies, continuance with postmenopausal estrogen therapy (ET) is associated with a reduction of 50% to 60% in the risk of osteoporosis-related hip fractures and of approximately 90% in that of vertebral fractures. The osteoporosis protective effect of ET was confirmed by the prospective Women's Health Initiative Study. Of 16,608 women aged 50 to 79 years who were randomized to receive ET (conjugated equine estrogen [CEE] 0.625 mg; medroxyprogesterone acetate [MPA] 5 mg) or placebo, the treated group had one third fewer hip fractures compared with the control group. The subjects who participated in this study were healthy postmenopausal women and were not prescreened for osteoporosis. As noted previously, osteoporotic fractures result from an interaction between:

- Reduced bone mass
- Disruption of the microarchitecture of the bone
- Falls and other minor trauma.

11

ET has a biologic action with respect to each of the above factors.

■ Mechanism of Action

Estrogen preserves bone mass for the following reasons:

- It is a potent antiresorptive agent that inhibits osteoclast activity, thereby reducing bone mineral loss.

- It stimulates collagen synthesis, a function of osteoblasts and the basis for osteoid formation, an essential step in bone mineralization (estrogen receptors are present in osteoclasts and osteoblasts) (Figure 2.7).
- It is essential for osteocyte recruitment and function. Osteocytes undergo apoptosis (cell death) in the presence of trabecular microdamage, with subsequent enhanced osteoclast (bone removal) activity.
- It enhances the absorption of calcium from the gastrointestinal tract.
- Estrogen stimulates the expression of the progesterone (Pa) gene via the estrogen receptor (ER)α and to a lesser extent ERβ activity.
- Current use of ET increases the mechanical strength of the proximal femur by improving its geometric properties.

Other postulated mechanisms of action include:
- Stimulation of calcitonin
- Modulation of parathyroid hormone (PTH) secretion
- An improvement in overall central nervous system (CNS) function, including balance, thus decreasing the likelihood of falls.

■ Dosage

The response of bone mineralization to estrogen therapy depends on the dose used. Previous studies have shown that a minimal plasma estradiol (E_2)level of 40 to 50 pg/mL must be maintained in order to prevent bone mineral loss and that a safe level to aim for is 60 pg/mL or higher. More recent data have confirmed that much lower doses of estrogen may be effective. The result depends on an individual's endogenous production of E_2, the level of sex hormone–binding globulin (SHBG) synthesized (and, therefore, the

190

amount of biologically active estrogen), and the patient's response to a given dose of estrogen. Figures 11.1, 11.2, and 11.3 illustrate these points:

- Serum E_2 levels >5 pg/dL in untreated, naturally postmenopausal women were associated with a significant decrease in the risk for vertebral and hip fracture compared with women with E_2 values <5 pg/dL (normal E_2 postmenopausal levels are <20 mg/dL). This is reflected in pretreatment lumbar spine BMD, as was recently confirmed by the author (Figure 11.2).

FIGURE 11.1 — SERUM ESTRADIOL CONCENTRATION AT BASELINE AND AGE-ADJUSTED RISK OF SUBSEQUENT HIP OR VERTEBRAL FRACTURE IN POSTMENOPAUSAL WOMEN

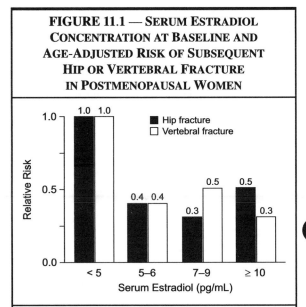

There were 317 women in the hip-fracture analysis and 282 in the vertebral-fracture analysis. The reference group consisted of the women with serum estradiol concentrations <5 pg/mL. To convert values for estradiol to picomoles per liter, multiply by 3.67. *P* for trend <0.01 for hip fracture and <0.005 for vertebral fracture.

Adapted from: Cummings SR, et al. *N Engl J Med.* 1998;339:735.

191

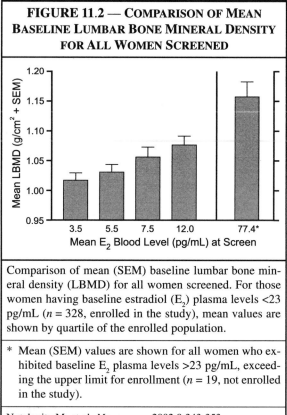

FIGURE 11.2 — COMPARISON OF MEAN BASELINE LUMBAR BONE MINERAL DENSITY FOR ALL WOMEN SCREENED

Comparison of mean (SEM) baseline lumbar bone mineral density (LBMD) for all women screened. For those women having baseline estradiol (E_2) plasma levels <23 pg/mL ($n = 328$, enrolled in the study), mean values are shown by quartile of the enrolled population.

* Mean (SEM) values are shown for all women who exhibited baseline E_2 plasma levels >23 pg/mL, exceeding the upper limit for enrollment ($n = 19$, not enrolled in the study).

Notelovitz M, et al. *Menopause*. 2002;9:343-353.

- The risk of fracture was substantially increased with SHBG levels (endogenous) above 1 µg/dL. The dose, type, and route of ET impacts on the hepatic synthesis of SHBG. In one study, 0.625 mg CEE increased SHBG concentrations by 100% after 3 to 4 months of therapy. Equivalent increases after 1 mg oral $17\beta E_2$ and 0.05 mg transdermal E_2 were 42% and 12%, respectively. Because of the hepatic first-pass effect of oral estrogen, approximately 40 times more

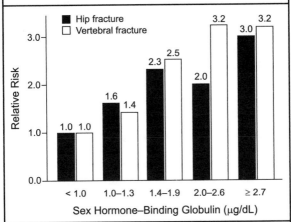

FIGURE 11.3 — SERUM CONCENTRATIONS OF SEX HORMONE–BINDING GLOBULIN AT BASELINE* AND AGE-ADJUSTED RISK OF SUBSEQUENT HIP OR VERTEBRAL FRACTURE IN POSTMENOPAUSAL WOMEN

There were 476 women in the hip-fracture analysis and 399 in the vertebral-fracture analysis. The reference group consisted of the women with values in the lowest quintile (<1.0 μg/dL). To convert values for sex hormone–binding globulin (SHBG) to nanomoles per liter, multiply by 34.7. P for trend <0.05 for hip fracture and <0.001 for vertebral fracture.

* In quintiles.

Adapted from: Cummings SR, et al. *N Engl J Med*. 1998;339:736.

estrogen has to be delivered in order to achieve equivalent levels of "free" E_2 after nonoral ET. Thus, a 1-mg dose $17\beta E_2$ is actually equivalent in terms of plasma free E_2 levels to 0.025 μg transdermal estrogen.

With the recent discovery of ERα and ERβ and their heterogeneic distribution in various estrogen-target tissues, the varied response of patients to a given dose of estrogen is predictable. ERα is the predominant isoform and its interaction with ERβ is influenced by the stage of osteoblast differentiation. Under certain circumstances, ERβ can inhibit the ERα activity in bone cells. This may explain (as illustrated in Figure 11.4) why for a given plasma E_2 level (eg, 20 pg/dL) following esterified estrogen therapy some patients will respond with a substantial increase in their bone mineral density (BMD), while others will lose BMD. Additional reasons include differences in the ability of osteoblasts to aromatize androgens to estrogen and so provide a direct local source of active estrogen for bone. Variations in the catabolic pathways that con-

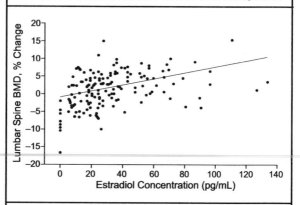

FIGURE 11.4 — LUMBAR SPINE* BMD PERCENTAGE OF CHANGE FROM BASELINE AT 24 MONTHS VS PLASMA ESTRADIOL CONCENTRATION FOR INDIVIDUAL SUBJECTS

The correlation is bone mineral density (BMD) percent change = 0.074 estradiol concentration − 1.13 ($R = 0.37$, $P = 0.001$, $n = 152$).

* L1 through L4.

Adapted from: Genant HK, et al. *Arch Intern Med*. 1997;157:2613.

vert estrone (E_1) to intermediate metabolites of variable estrogenic activity are also relevant. Hydroxylation of E_1 to the D-ring metabolites (16 OHE$_1$ and estriol) will retain proestrogenic activity. Metabolism via the A-ring will result in the predominance of the 2-hydroxyestrogens (OHE$_1$ and 2 methoxy estrogens), which are almost devoid of estrogenic activity. These two pathways are mutually exclusive. These new findings have consolidated the author's practice of adjustive hormone therapy (HT)—adjusting the dose of estrogen according to the need and response of the patient over time (Figure 11.5 and Table 11.1). The objective is to prescribe a dose of estrogen sufficient to raise the BMD into a protective range and then to gradually titrate the dose downward to maintain the BMD and to meet the other HT needs of the patient. This will vary with the patient's endogenous synthesis of estrogen and androgen and the bioavailability of the steroids. Table 11.2 lists available hormonal preparations.

To maintain bone mass, the following dose-equivalents are useful in treating symptomatic post-menopausal women with normal to low-normal bone mass (mild osteopenia equivalent to 1 to 2 standard deviations [SD] below normal young adult values):

- Estrace (micronized 17βE$_2$): 0.5 mg/day
- Estraderm (17βE$_2$): 0.05 mg-patch biweekly; Vivelle 0.025-mg to 0.05 mg-patch biweekly; Climara 0.025-mg, 0.05 mg-patch weekly; Alora 0.025-mg to 0.05-mg patch biweekly
- Ethinyl estradiol: 5 µg/day
- Ogen (estropipate): 0.625 mg/day
- Premarin (CEE): 0.625 mg/day. Lower doses of CEE, 0.45 mg and 0.3 mg, have been found to be equally effective.

The above doses of estrogen should be complemented with a total of 1500 mg/day of elemental calcium.

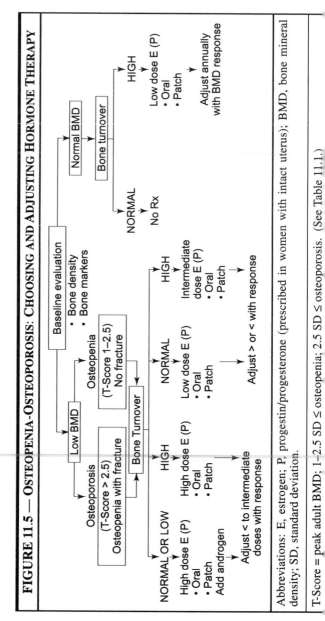

FIGURE 11.5 — OSTEOPENIA-OSTEOPOROSIS: CHOOSING AND ADJUSTING HORMONE THERAPY

Abbreviations: E, estrogen; P, progestin/progesterone (prescribed in women with intact uterus); BMD, bone mineral density; SD, standard deviation.

T-Score = peak adult BMD; 1–2.5 SD ≤ osteopenia; 2.5 SD ≤ osteoporosis. (See Table 11.1.)

TABLE 11.1 — OSTEOPENIA-OSTEOPOROSIS: CHOOSING AND ADJUSTING THE DOSE OF ESTROGEN			
Estrogen	**Low**	**Intermediate**	**High**
17β-estradiol	0.5 mg	1 mg	2 mg
CEE	0.3 mg	0.625 mg	0.9 mg
Estradiol patch	25 μg	50 μg	100 μg
Abbreviation: CEE, conjugated equine estrogen.			
See Figure 11.5.			

It should be noted that although the majority of women on maintenance doses of ET will not lose BMD, approximately 30% to 40% of women on the ultra-low doses of ET (0.025-mg patch; 0.5 mg oral $17\beta E_2$) will continue to lose bone mass. Patients on ultra-low doses of ET should be closely monitored (Figure 11.6).

To increase bone mass in patients with moderate-to-severe osteopenia (BMD $\geq$2 SD below young adult normal values) or with documented osteoporosis, one of the following dose-equivalent estrogens should be prescribed:

- Estrace (micronized $17\beta E_2$): 1 or 2 mg/day
- Estraderm ($17\beta E_2$ patch): 0.1 mg biweekly; Vivelle 0.75 to 0.1 mg biweekly; Climara 0.05 mg, 0.1 mg weekly; Alora 0.75 to 0.1 mg biweekly
- Ethinyl estradiol: 10 to 20 μg/day
- Ogen (estropipate): 1.25 mg/day
- Premarin (CEE): 0.625 or 0.9 mg/day.

Estrogen therapy should be prescribed on a continuous basis. If side effects occur (eg, mastalgia), try a Monday-through-Friday regimen.

11

TABLE 11.2 — POSTMENOPAUSAL HORMONAL PREPARATIONS

Brand Name	Type of Hormone	Available Doses (mg)	Manufacturer
ORAL ESTROGENS			
Cenestin	Synthetic conjugated estrogens	0.3, 0.625, 0.9, 1.25	Duramed
Estrace	Micronized estradiol	0.5, 1, 2	Warner-Chilcott
Menest	Esterified estrogens	0.3, 0.625, 1.25, 2.5	Monarch
Ogen	Estropipate	0.625, 1.25, 2.5	Pharmacia & Upjohn
Ortho-Est	Estropipate	0.625, 1.25	Women First
Premarin	Conjugated equine estrogens	0.3, 0.625, 0.9, 1.25, 2.5	Wyeth
PARENTERAL ESTROGENS (injections, pellets, patches)			
Alora	Transdermal estradiol	0.025, 0.05, 0.075, 0.1	Watson
Climara	Transdermal estradiol	0.025, 0.05, 0.075, 0.1	Berlex
Estraderm	Transdermal estradiol	0.05, 0.1	Novartis
Vivelle	Transdermal estradiol	0.0375, 0.05, 0.075, 0.1	Novartis

PROGESTOGENS			
Aygestin	Norethindrone acetate	5	Wyeth
Megestrol acetate	Megestrol acetate	20, 40	Par, Roxane
Nor-QD	Norethindrone	0.35	Watson
Ortho Micronor	Norethindrone	0.35	Ortho-McNeil
Ovrette	Norgestrel	0.075	Wyeth
Provera	Medroxyprogesterone acetate	2.5, 5, 10	Pharmacia & Upjohn
PROGESTERONES			
Prometrium	Micronized oral progesterone	100	Solvay
Crinone	Progesterone vaginal suppositories	4%, 8%	Serono
ORAL ANDROGENS			
Android	Methyltestosterone	10	ICN
Halotestin	Fluoxymesterone	5, 10	Pharmacia & Upjohn
Testred	Methyltestosterone	10	ICN
Virilon	Methyltestosterone	10	Star

11

Continued

Brand Name	Type of Hormone	Available Doses (mg)	Manufacturer
INJECTABLE ANDROGENS			
Delatestryl	Testosterone enanthate	200 mg/mL	BTG
ESTROGEN/ANDROGEN or PROGESTOGEN COMBINATIONS			
Activella	Estradiol/norethindrone acetate	1 / 0.5	Pharmacia & Upjohn
CombiPatch	Estradiol/norethindrone acetate	0.05 / 0.14, 0.05 / 0.25	Novartis
Estratest	Esterified estrogens/methyltestosterone	1.25 / 2.5	Solvay
Estratest H.S.	Esterified estrogens/methyltestosterone	0.625 / 1.25	Solvay
Femhrt	Ethinyl estradiol/norethindrone acetate	5 µg / 1 mg	Parke-Davis
Ortho-Prefest	Estradiol/norgestimate	1 / 1 mg-0.09 mg	Monarch
Prempro	Conjugated estrogens/MPA	0.625 / 2.5, 0.625 / 5	Wyeth
Premphase	Conjugated estrogens/MPA	0.625 / 5	Wyeth
Abbreviation: MPA, medroxyprogesterone acetate.			

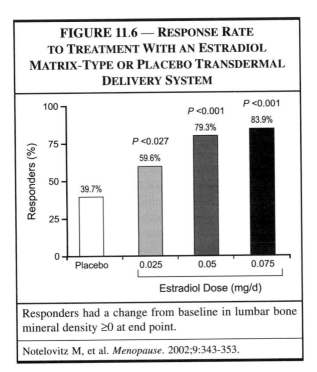

FIGURE 11.6 — RESPONSE RATE TO TREATMENT WITH AN ESTRADIOL MATRIX-TYPE OR PLACEBO TRANSDERMAL DELIVERY SYSTEM

Responders had a change from baseline in lumbar bone mineral density ≥0 at end point.

Notelovitz M, et al. *Menopause*. 2002;9:343-353.

■ Nonresponse to Estrogen Therapy

Some patients do not respond to oral estrogens because of:

- Gastrointestinal (GI) side effects (often caused by the lactose "filler")
- Malabsorption or nonabsorption
- The enterohepatic binding of estrogen.

Nonresponders are identified by:

- Loss of BMD despite "adequate" oral estrogen therapy
- Increase in the urine calcium-to-creatinine ratio with appropriate calculated calcium intake
- Increase in urinary collagen cross-link excretion

- Suboptimal plasma E_2 and/or E_1 levels
- Plasma estrogen consistent with the oral dose of estrogen but with increased plasma follicle-stimulating hormone (FSH) levels, indicating possible "estrogen binding." In premenopausal women, the negative feedback on the pituitary synthesis of FSH is mediated via both E_2 and inhibin B. The latter is absent in postmenopausal women. Exogenous ET will, in a dose-response manner, decrease postmenopausal elevations in FSH, but the response will be blunted or remain in the low menopausal range: 40-50 min/mL. FSH levels in the premenopausal range (<20 min/mL) are indicative of estrogen excess.
- No relief of vasomotor symptoms.

Alternative treatments include:
- Conversion to oral $17\beta E_2$ if the patient is being treated with CEE
- $17\beta E_2$ patches: 0.1 mg 2 times weekly (or its equivalent)
- Estrogen pellets ($17\beta E_2$): 25 to 50 mg subcutaneously every 6 months
- Adding androgen or an androgenic progestin (see Chapter 13).

■ Starting Estrogen Therapy

Bone mineral is lost at the rate of 1% to 3% per year during the first 5 to 6 years after the last menstrual period. Recent data have confirmed that women over 65 years of age continue to lose BMD.

A recent study has shown that in physically frail elderly women (>75 years of age), there is a significant increase in the BMD of the lumbar spine and hip following combination HT. It should be considered on a selective basis. BMD testing provides objective indications for early estrogen therapy. Early treatment is indicated for the following women:

- Premature/surgically menopausal women, especially if below the age of 40
- Women with a BMD ≥ 1 SD below normal young adult values
- Bone density loss >1%/year on repeated BMD testing
- Persistent increase in the early morning urine calcium-to-creatinine ratio (>0.16) and/or excess urinary excretion of cross-linked collagen
- Women at high risk, such as those who have:
  - Family history of osteoporosis
  - Premenopausal oligomenorrhea or amenorrhea
  - Late menarche — after 16 years of age
  - Athletic amenorrhea
  - Low body fat — <20% of total body weight
  - Anovulatory cycles
- Patients with other medical problems, such as:
  - Malabsorption syndrome
  - GI bypass procedures
  - Asthmatics on steroid therapy
  - Hyperthyroidism
  - Patients on thyroid replacement therapy.

11

NOTE: Oral contraceptives have a bone-protective effect and in some high-performance exercisers have increased bone density by 9.5%. The use of low-dose preparations (eg, in the United States—Ovcon-35, Nordette, Desogen, Loestrin 21; in Canada—Marvelon, Min-Ovral, Ortho-Cept) should result in improvement in bone mass. Long-term use of depot MPA may be associated with a significant decrease in BMD. Women who use depot MPA before they reach their peak bone mass and/or those on long-term treatment may be especially vulnerable.

It is never too late to start treatment. Studies have confirmed that osteopenic women >65 years of age and women with established osteoporosis increase their BMD with estrogen therapy.

The same dosages are used in older women, although they may be more sensitive to estrogen. If sensitivity occurs, decrease the dose one level, or prescribe on a Monday-through-Friday schedule.

■ How Long to Treat?

Estrogen therapy for osteoporosis prevention and management should last a minimum of 10 to 15 years and probably should be lifelong in the absence of side effects. Bone mass is lost rapidly when estrogen therapy is stopped and may reach pretreatment levels within 4 years of stopping treatment.

■ Monitoring Estrogen Therapy

Estrogen therapy needs to be monitored annually for efficacy and safety:

- Efficacy:
  - Repeat dual-energy x-ray absorptiometry (DEXA) or other BMD testing
  - Urine calcium-to-creatinine ratio
  - Urine collagen cross-links, for example Osteomark (N-telopeptide) or Pyrilinks-D
  - Alkaline phosphatase (bone-specific, if available)
  - Selectively—plasma E_2, E_1, and FSH levels. Pretreatment measurement of E_2 is gaining more acceptance. The recent commercial availability of high-sensitivity and specific E_2 assays has documented the wide variation of endogenous E_2 synthesis. The ability to ad-

just the dose of ET according to the patient's baseline plasma E_2 and clinical need is now feasible and practical. For this reason, the author favors E_2-based preparations since posttreatment assays are more reflective of the ET prescribed.

- Safety:
  - Annual breast examination and mammogram. Particular attention should be given to women with increased mammographic density pretreatment. Women with dense breasts on mammography are at increased risk of breast cancer. Dense breasts may reflect increased endogenous breast tissue estrogen synthesis
  - Endometrial monitoring:
    - Annual endometrial biopsy if on ET alone
    - Vaginal ultrasound if on combination hormone therapy
    - If endometrial thickness exceeds 5 mm on ultrasound, endometrial biopsy.

For endometrial biopsies, use the least invasive technique, such as Pipelle or Gyno-Sampler endometrial aspirators.

Progestogens and Progesterone 11

Progestogens and progesterone are prescribed for one reason only: to protect the endometrium. Progesterone receptors are, however, present in osteoblasts. Based on *in vivo* and clinical studies, it is now believed that progesterone may stimulate new bone formation, although the mechanism has not been identified. Premenopausal women with anovulatory, but regular, cycles have reduced bone mass.

■ Type and Dose of Progestogen/Progesterone

The type and dose of progestogen with maximal bone-stimulating effects has not as yet been identified, but clinical studies suggest that testosterone-derived progestogens (eg, norethindrone acetate [NETA]) have a greater anabolic effect on bone when combined with estrogen than either progesterone or progesterone-derived progestogen (eg, MPA). In one recent study, 1 mg NETA added to either 5 μg or 10 μg ethinyl estradiol (FemHRT), substantially increased the BMD response compared with that in the estrogen-alone–treated patients. The same was noted when 1 mg $17\beta E_2$ is added to 0.5 mg norethindrone (Activella). Progestogens/progesterone (in combination with estrogens) are prescribed in accepted endometrium-protecting and bleeding-control doses (Table 11.2). Micronized progesterone (Prometrium) is Food and Drug Administration (FDA) approved for use in HT.

■ Cyclic vs Continuous Combined Hormone Therapy (HT)

All hormonal regimens improve BMD equally well. The decision should be based on:

- *Patient compliance*: Women on cyclic progestogens will have monthly withdrawal bleeding; women on continuous combined therapy may have breakthrough bleeding for 4 to 6 months before becoming amenorrheic. Withdrawal bleeding is one of the primary reasons why women stop HT. This is less troublesome to perimenopausal and recently menopausal women than it is to those who have been amenorrheic for 5 or more years. Patients should be informed about what to expect before starting treatment.

- *Other medical indications*: Progestogens may decrease the lipid-lowering effect of estrogen, may induce insulin-peripheral resistance, and may increase risk of vasospasm. This is more likely to occur with MPA and least likely with micronized progesterone or NETA. The latter—but not progesterone—lowers HDL-cholesterol. NETA, but not progesterone, decreases plasma triglycerides. Thus the selection of a progestogen should be governed not only by the presence of dyslipidemia but the type of abnormality. Progestogens can be used to advantage therapeutically provided the patients are tested before therapy. This requires a fasting lipid profile. Patients at high risk of cardiovascular disease (ie, women with hyperlipidemia, diabetes, or hypertension) should be given low-dose NETA or preferably micronized progesterone cyclically rather than continuously. This is also true for women with migraine headaches.

■ Progestogen/Progesterone Regimens

- *Cyclic*:
  - Provera (MPA): 5 or 10 mg, day 1 through day 12 or 14 of the month
  - Colprone (medrogestone): 5 or 10 mg, day 1 through day 12 or 14
  - Aygestin (NETA): 1 mg, day 1 through day 12 or 14
  - Micronized progesterone: 200 mg in the evening, day 1 through day 12 or 14
- *Continuous*:
  - Provera (MPA): 2.5 mg/day
  - Aygestin (NETA): 1.25 mg/day

11

- Ortho Micronor (norethindrone): 35 µg two
    to three tablets daily
- Nor-QD (35 µg per tablet): two tablets daily
- Micronized progesterone: 100 mg/day
- *Intermittent.*

Controlled, 1-year studies have shown that 2 weeks of progestogen therapy every 3 months is as effective as monthly cyclic progestogens in preventing endometrial hyperplasia. Although the study results need to be confirmed, this approach may be useful in women who would benefit from cyclic progestogen, but are reluctant to have monthly periods. Use the same dose listed under *Cyclic* section.

NOTE: Estrogen simulates progesterone receptors. An appropriate dose of estrogen is mandatory when treating postmenopausal women; otherwise, progestogen will not be effective. The dose of progestogen will depend on the amount of estrogen used. Fortunately, the dose of progestogen needed for bleeding control appears to be optimal for bone remodeling as well.

■ Who Should Receive Progestogen?

The following women should receive progestogen in addition to estrogen:

- Women with an intact uterus
- Because of its anabolic effects, progestogens can be considered in all women with BMDs 3 SD below normal young adult values. This may also be appropriate for women who have had a hysterectomy (NETA is the progestogen recommended). The androgenic progestogens lower SHBG significantly and in so doing may make both endogenous estrogens and androgens, as well as the estrogen prescribed, more bioavailable

- Progesterone blocks the glucocorticoid receptor in bone. Women on long-term corticosteroids (asthmatics and those with arthritis) should be considered for combination estrogen/progestogen therapy.

■ Safety

Progestogens are safe. Some women have side effects, mainly:
- Mood change
- Irritability
- Depression.

If side effects occur, reduce the dose and/or change the type of progestogen, for example, from MPA to norethindrone or natural progesterone. In rare instances of sensitivity to all systemic progestogens/progesterone, consider using a progesterone-medicated intrauterine device (IUD), such as the levonorgestrel-containing Mirena IUD.

Progestogens are not approved by the FDA for the prevention and/or treatment of osteoporosis.

Androgens

Data in women are limited, but androgens have been shown to decrease bone turnover in postmenopausal women. Preliminary studies show that estrogen-androgen combinations enhance bone mass to a greater extent than estrogen-alone treatment. Estrogen/androgen therapy is currently indicated for the treatment of moderate-to-severe vasomotor symptoms not improved by estrogens alone and is not FDA-approved for the prevention and/or treatment of osteoporosis. However, there is a sound biologic rationale for the use of estrogen/androgen therapy in the treatment of women with osteoporosis.

Estrone and estradiol are derived from androgens (androstenedione and testosterone, respectively) in both premenopausal and postmenopausal women (Figure 11.7). The bioavailable androgens are:

- DHEAS (not shown in Figure 11.7 and derived primarily from the adrenal gland)
- DHEA
- Androstenedione
- Testosterone; the latter three androgens are synthesized in almost equal proportions from the adrenal gland and ovarian stroma.

The androgen/estrogen metabolic pathway is mediated by various enzymes: aromatase, 17β-hydroxysteroid dehydrogenase, sulfatase — all of which are genetically programmed and controlled. Testosterone exerts its effect via specific testosterone binding receptors present in the three main bone cell types (osteoclasts, osteocytes, and osteoblasts) or via its bioconversion to either E_2 or by 5α-reductase activity, to the most potent androgen: dihydrotestosterone (DHT). The bone cells have receptors for DHEA, DHT, and E_2. The amount of androgen synthesized relative to estrogen is summarized in Table 11.3.

Androgen enhances osteoblast differentiation and the synthesis of the extracellular matrix proteins such as type $1\alpha1$ collagen, osteocalcin, and osteonectin. Androgens also stimulate mineralization, and they influence the bone cell's function through their effect on local and systemic factors that control the bone cell's microenvironment.

Often overlooked is the effect of androgens on muscle physiology. As noted previously, there are clear associations between muscle mass, muscle strength, and bone density. Approximately 4% of muscle mass is lost during the first 3 years after menopause. Muscle strength is lost earlier in women than in men and may account for their greater tendency to fall. Because muscle strength is lost first in the upper extremities and precedes bone loss, a grip-strength test is a good predictor of future lower extremity bone loss and balance problems. Post-

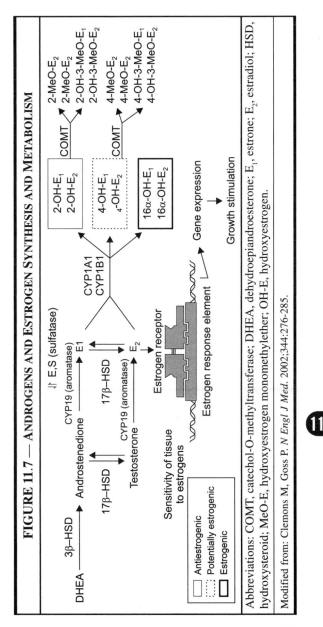

FIGURE 11.7 — ANDROGENS AND ESTROGEN SYNTHESIS AND METABOLISM

Abbreviations: COMT, catechol-O-methyltransferase; DHEA, dehydroepiandrosterone; E_1, estrone; E_2, estradiol; HSD, hydroxysteroid; MeO-E, hydroxyestrogen monomethylether; OH-E, hydroxyestrogen.

Modified from: Clemons M, Goss P. *N Engl J Med.* 2002;344:276-285.

TABLE 11.3 — MEAN STEROID LEVELS IN WOMEN

	Reproductive Age (pg/mL)	Natural Menopause (pg/mL)	Surgical Menopause (pg/mL)
Estradiol	150	10-15	10
Testosterone	400	290	110
Androstenedione	1900	1000	700
DHEA	5000	2000	1800
DHEAS	3,000,000	1,000,000	1,000,000

Abbreviations: DHEA, dehydroepiandrosterone; DHEAS, dehydroepiandrosterone sulfate.

Adapted from: Lobo RA. *Treatment of Postmenopausal Women: Basic and Clinical Aspects.* Boston, Mass: Lippincott Williams & Wilkins. 1999; and Judd HL, et al. *J Clin Endocrinol Metab.* 1974;39:1020-1024.

menopausal androgen therapy increases lean tissue mass and decreases fat mass. A recent double-blind randomized study evaluated body composition (by DEXA) and muscle strength (by comparing the repetition maximum [RM] in separate arm and leg bench-press exercises). As shown in Table 11.4, women treated with estrogen/androgen therapy (esterified estrogen 1.25 mg; methyltestosterone 2.5 mg) compared with estrogen-alone therapy (esterified estrogen 1.25 mg) had a significant increase in their lean tissue mass and a comparable improvement in lower body muscle strength. The serum values of free testosterone (a measure of endogenous androgens) were significantly greater in the androgen-supplemented group compared with the estrogen-alone treatment group. SHBG values were also significantly lower in the estrogen/androgen group.

Androgens are rarely prescribed alone. Available androgens are listed in Table 11.2. Typical regimens include:

- *Oral*:
  - Estratest (esterified estrogen [ESE] 1.25 mg and methyltestosterone 2.5 mg): one tablet daily
  - Estratest H.S. (ESE 0.625 mg and methyltestosterone 1.25 mg): one tablet daily
- *Parenteral*:
  - Testosterone pellets, 50 mg, and E_2 implants 25 to 50 mg, every 6 months
  - Testosterone propionate or enanthate injectable, 75 mg intramuscularly (IM) every 6 to 8 weeks (not recommended)
  - A testosterone patch is being developed but is not yet clinically available.

■ **Who Should Receive Androgens**?

Until more information is available, estrogen/androgen combinations should be used selectively in

TABLE 11.4 — CHANGE IN LEAN TISSUE MASS AND STRENGTH AFTER ESTROGEN OR ESTROGEN/ANDROGEN THERAPY

	Pre-E	Post-E	Pre-E/A	Post-E/A	P-value
Lean tissue (kg)					
Upper	1.91	1.94	1.90	2.08	<0.02
Trunk	20.58	20.61	20.48	21.29	<0.001
Lower	6.85	6.91	6.77	7.01	<0.04
Muscle strength (lb)					
Lower body press	232	257	235	286	<0.002

Estrogen/androgen (E/A) greater in free-T and greater decrease in sex hormone–binding globulin compared with estrogen (E) only.

Dobs AS, et al. *J Clin Endocr Metab.* 2002;87:1509-1516.

women with BMDs ≥2.5 to 3 SD below normal young adult values, particularly if they are not responsive to estrogen monotherapy, and especially in surgically menopausal women. An additional indication for combined estrogen/androgen therapy is in patients with elevated triglycerides who require hormone therapy. The addition of methyltestosterone will significantly decrease triglyceride levels without compromising the rest of the lipid profile except for high-density lipoprotein (HDL) cholesterol. For women with normal pretreatment HDL-cholesterol levels, this decrease in HDL cholesterol will not be clinically relevant. Women with pretreatment HDL-cholesterol values <35 mg/dL should not be given synthetic androgens but can be treated safely with "natural" testosterone.

All women with an intact uterus require added progestogens as androgens do not protect against estrogen-induced endometrial hyperplasia. Micronized progesterone is the preferred drug.

■ **Safety**

Side effects include:

• Oily skin
• Hair growth
• Voice change (may be permanent).

If a patient is being treated with natural testosterone, monitor plasma testosterone and free testosterone values every 6 months. Methyltestosterone is not measurable with standard testosterone assays. Women with low HDL cholesterol should be monitored every 3 to 6 months. The added estrogen usually compensates for the potential HDL cholesterol–lowering effect of synthetic androgens.

■ Breast Cancer and Estrogen Therapy

Despite over 40 observational studies, there is still no consensus on breast cancer risk with ET, and most authorities agree that estrogen may be a promoter rather than a cause of breast cancer. The relative risk of breast cancer for ET-treated women appears to be time dependent and increases by 30% to 40% after 10 to 15 years of ET. A similar result was noted in the recent Women's Health Initiative Study (WHI). The relative risk may also be dose dependent. In absolute terms, the actual number of women who will develop (but not die from) breast cancer increases from 45 cases of breast cancer per 1000 untreated women aged 50 to 70 years to 47 per 1000 and 51 per 1000 for women treated with HT for 5 and 10 years, respectively. Women not taking HT have a greater chance of dying from breast cancer than do ET-treated women. One study places the benefit/risk ratio of ET in perspective (Figure 11.8). Although more women die from breast cancer than heart disease in the perimenopausal years, deaths from cardiovascular disease postmenopause far exceed deaths from both breast and lung cancer. Although contested by the recent WHI study, over 30 observational studies have shown ET reduces cardiovascular disease by 50% if therapy is started early.

■ The HERS Study

In the Heart and Estrogen/Progestin Replacement Study (HERS), the use of CEE and MPA (Prempro) in women with significant and serious cardiovascular disease resulted in no protection against myocardial infarction and/or coronary heart disease (CHD) death when compared with a matched group not on HT. Both groups were on a multiplicity of drugs for the treatment of their heart disease. Although a number of statistically related reasons for these results have been

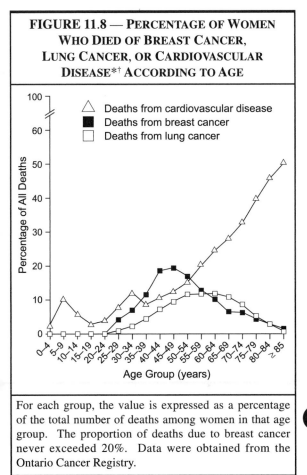

FIGURE 11.8 — PERCENTAGE OF WOMEN WHO DIED OF BREAST CANCER, LUNG CANCER, OR CARDIOVASCULAR DISEASE*† ACCORDING TO AGE

For each group, the value is expressed as a percentage of the total number of deaths among women in that age group. The proportion of deaths due to breast cancer never exceeded 20%. Data were obtained from the Ontario Cancer Registry.

* Includes cerebrovascular causes.
† In Ontario in 1995.

Adapted from: Phillips KA, et al. *N Engl J Med*. 1999;340:143.

suggested (see references), the following important clinical points may help guide clinical practice:

- Estrogen-alone therapy—CEE 0.625 mg—has been shown to improve the survival of treated vs nontreated women in at least four studies of women with angiographic evidence of 50% to 75% stenosis of their coronary arteries. This does not infer that ET will reverse the degree of plaque formation or stenosis, but ET could improve the function of the diseased coronary artery, subject to the following additional three caveats.

- Animal studies have clearly demonstrated that MPA—and not natural progesterone or NETA—antagonizes estrogen's ability to decrease plaque formation in coronary arteries and to significantly reduce estrogen-induced vasodilation of the coronary arteries.

- Reduced bioavailable estradiol in susceptible individuals. CEE stimulates three times as much SHBG as equivalent doses of micronized estradiol or estradiol valerate. The concentration of ER decreases significantly in diseased vs healthy coronary arteries.

- The type of plaque. Those with a fibrous capsule are resistant to fracture. Fatty plaques are most likely to be disrupted and encourage thrombus formation with luminal obstruction.

■ Women's Health Initiative Study

The WHI was conceived as a primary prevention trial to establish whether estrogen alone or estrogen plus a progestogen could reduce the risk of cardiovascular disease (CVD) in healthy postmenopausal women. The study found a small excess in cases of breast cancer, myocardial infarction, cerebrovascular accident, and venous thrombosis in conjunction with a small decrease in the number of cases of bone fracture and colon cancer. In the author's opinion, this study and the resulting conclusions were flawed by at least three major misconceptions:

- That all menopausal women have the same hormonal (and other) biology
- That women aged 60+ years are free of coronary artery atherosclerosis
- That CEE and MPA are representative of all other HTs.

The only feature truly common to all menopausal women is cessation of menstruation. The polymorphism of the various organ sex-steroid receptors is variable between and within individuals, as is the genetic control of their hormonal synthesis and metabolism. Giving all women a "standard" dose of estrogen/progestogen will result in an unknown number of women being either undertreated or overtreated.

As shown in Figure 11.9, the pathogenesis of atherosclerosis (as with osteoporosis) commences in early adolescence. By the time women in Western societies reach the age of menopause, most if not all have a variable degree of atherogenic disease (albeit silent). Primary CVD prevention is a premenopausal practice; selective HT is appropriate for secondary intervention in perimenopausal women without overt CVD (as opposed to prevention). Treating older postmenopausal women without close clinical evaluation could expose a few (who have the same metabolic profile as the women who experienced adverse CVD events in the WHI study) to a cardiac event. However, the vast majority will not suffer any ill effects.

Nonpregnant women synthesize only two bioavailable estrogens (Figure 11.7): E_1 and E_2. The amount produced and their catabolic pathways (as noted earlier) are highly variable and can impact significantly (either positively or negatively) on conditions such as CVD, osteoporosis, and breast cancer.

FIGURE 11.9 — TIMELINE REDEFINING DISEASE PREVENTION AND HEALTH PROMOTION INTERVENTION

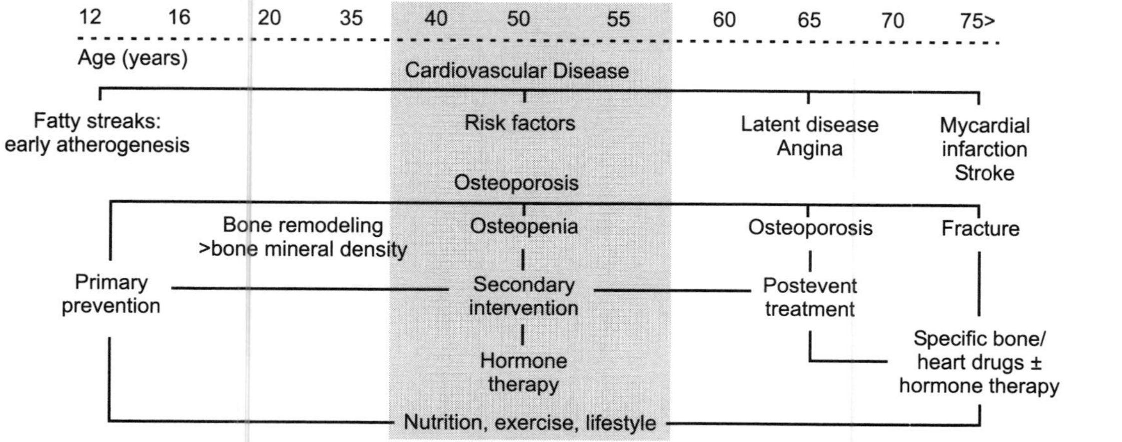

Shaded area represents the window of therapeutic opportunity for estrogen therapy–associated cardiovascular disease and bone protection.

The use of CEE, although a safe and effective form of estrogen, does have unique pharmacokinetics and pharmacokinetic actions that differ from that of E_2. Also, MPA has certain unique properties that may be of disadvantage to women with asymptomatic or overt atherosclerosis, such as:

- A prolonged half-life of 20+ hours (progestogens down-regulate estrogen receptors)
- Antagonism of the antiatherogenic effect of estrogen
- Enhancement of coronary artery smooth muscle
- Up-regulation of thrombin receptor expression (and hence an increased risk of thrombosis)
- Potentiation of endothelin 1 and coronary artery vasoconstriction.

None of the patients with reported adverse events died. The actual risk was also small: 37 HT-treated women vs 30 placebo-treated women had coronary heart events annually for 10,000 women studied. A similar minority of women were adversely affected when risk of HT-related breast cancer was examined: 35 vs 30 events annually for 10,000 women on HT and placebo, respectively. Although these figures could be extrapolated to involve many women if applied to the nation, clinical decisions are made based on the profile and needs of the individual patient. This serves as the basis for the author's approach to HT (Table 11.5).

■ Clinical Application: CVD and HT

For women with known or suspected CVD (and in whom there is an indication for HT), the author recommends prescribing natural estrogen in a dose that will achieve a plasma E_2 of 60 pg/dL (total: endogenous + exogenous E_2) with a minimal increase in SHBG. Only natural micronized progesterone should be used for endometrial protection in a cyclic dose of 200 mg HS from day 1 through day 12 of each month.

Depending on the age of the patient, a progesterone/progestogen IUD should be considered, thus avoiding all systemic progesterone/progestin therapy.

Summary

A guide to HT and suggestions for tailoring the prescription are shown in Table 11.5.

TABLE 11.5 — OSTEOPOROSIS AND ADJUSTIVE HORMONE THERAPY: TAILORING THE PRESCRIPTION

- Hormone therapy needs to be tailored to the individual patient's needs. This includes other indications for hormone therapy, such as symptom relief.
- Patients who require bone mineral density maintenance need a lower dose of estrogen than those with osteoporosis.
- Women with marked osteopenia will benefit from added androgenic progestogens and androgens.
- Long-term treatment and, therefore, compliance are essential. Choose progestogen regimens that are acceptable to the patient.
- Monitor progress by regular assessments, preferably by some method of bone mineral density measurement together with urine calcium-to-creatinine ratio and urine collagen cross-links testing.
- Reevaluate the type, dose, and route of administration of hormone therapy annually, and adjust accordingly.

SUGGESTED READING

Abdalla HI, Hart DM, Lindsay R, Leggate I, Hooke A. Prevention of bone mineral loss in postmenopausal women by norethisterone. *Obstet Gynecol.* 1985;66:789-792.

Albagha OM, McGuigan FE, Reid DM, Ralston SH. Estrogen receptor alpha gene polymorphisms and bone mineral density: haplotype analysis in women from the United Kingdom. *J Bone Miner Res.* 2001;16:128-134.

Barrett-Connor E, Wenger NK, Grady D, et al. Coronary heart disease in women, randomized clinical trials, HERS and RUTH. *Maturitas.* 1998;31:1-7.

Barzel US. Osteoporosis: taking a fresh look. *Hosp Pract.* 1996;31:59-68.

Beck TJ, Stone KL, Oreskovic TL, et al. Effects of current and discontinued estrogen replacement therapy on hip structural geometry: The Study of Osteoporotic Fractures. *J Bone Miner Res.* 2001;16:2103-2110.

Bemben DA, Langdon DB. Relationship between estrogen use and musculoskeletal function in postmenopausal women. *Maturitas.* 2002;42:119-127.

Berenson AB, Radecki CM, Grady JJ, Rickert VI, Thomas A. A prospective, controlled study of the effects of hormonal contraception on bone mineral density. *Obstet Gynecol.* 2001;98:576-582.

Bilezikian JP. Sex steroids, mice, and men: when androgens and estrogens get very close to each other. *J Bone Miner Res.* 2002;17:563-566.

Burkman RT Jr. Noncontraceptive effects of hormonal contraceptives: bone mass, sexually transmitted disease and pelvic inflammatory disease, cardiovascular disease, menstrual function, and future fertility. *Am J Obstet Gynecol.* 1994;170: 1569-1575.

Chen TL, Aronow L, Feldman D. Glucocorticoid receptors and inhibition of bone cell growth in primary culture. *Endocrinology.* 1977;100:619-628.

11

Christiansen C, Christensen MS, Transbol I. Bone mass in post-menopausal women after withdrawal of oestrogen/gestagen replacement therapy. *Lancet*. 1981;1:459-461.

Christensen MS, Hagen C, Christiansen C, Transbol I. Dose-response evaluation of cyclic estrogen/gestagen in postmenopausal women: placebo-controlled trial of its gynecologic and metabolic actions. *Am J Obstet Gynecol*. 1982;144:873-879.

Christiansen C, Lindsay R. Estrogens, bone loss and preservation. *Osteoporos Int*. 1990;1:7-13.

Christiansen C, Riis BJ. 17ß-estradiol and continuous norethisterone: a unique treatment for established osteoporosis in elderly women. *J Clin Endocrinol Metab*. 1990;71:836-841.

Collaborative Group on Hormonal Factors in Breast Cancer. Breast cancer and hormone replacement therapy: collaborative reanalysis of data from 51 epidemiological studies of 52,705 women with breast cancer and 108,411 women without breast cancer. *Lancet*. 1997;350:1047-1059.

Cummings SR, Browner WS, Bauer D, et al. Endogenous hormones and the risk of hip and vertebral fractures among older women. Study of Osteoporotic Fractures Research Group. *N Engl J Med*. 1998;339:733-738.

Cundy T, Cornish J, Roberts H, Elder H, Reid IR. Spinal bone density in women using depot medroxyprogesterone contraception. *Obstet Gynecol*. 1998;92(pt 1):569-573.

De Crée C, Lewin R, Ostyn M. Suitability of cyproterone acetate in the treatment of osteoporosis associated with athletic amenorrhea. *Int J Sports Med*. 1988;9:187-192.

Delmas PD. Treatment of postmenopausal osteoporosis. *Lancet*. 2002;359:2018-2026.

Dobs AS, Nguyen T, Pace C, Roberts CP. Differential effects of oral estrogen versus oral estrogen-androgen replacement therapy on body composition in postmenopausal women. *J Clin Endocrinol Metab*. 2002;87:1509-1516.

Dupont WD, Page DL. Menopausal estrogen replacement therapy and breast cancer. *Arch Intern Med*. 1991;151:67-72.

Eriksen EF, Colvard DS, Berg NJ, et al. Evidence of estrogen receptors in normal human osteoblast-like cells. *Science*. 1988;241: 84-86.

Ettinger B, Genant HK, Cann CE. Long-term estrogen replacement therapy prevents bone loss and fractures. *Ann Intern Med*. 1985;102:319-324.

Ettinger B, Genant HK, Cann CE. Low-dosage estrogen combined with calcium prevents postmenopausal bone loss: results of a three-year study. In: Cohn DV, Martin TJ, Meunier PJ, eds. *Calcium Regulation and Bone Metabolism: Basic and Clinical Aspects*. Amsterdam: Elsevier; 1987:918-922.

Ettinger B, Genant HK, Steiger P, Madvig P. Low-dosage micronized 17ß-estradiol prevents bone loss in postmenopausal women. *Am J Obstet Gynecol*. 1992;166:479-488.

Felson DT, Zhang Y, Hannan MT, Kiel DP, Wilson PW, Anderson JJ. The effect of postmenopausal estrogen therapy on bone density in elderly women. *N Engl J Med*. 1993;329:1141-1146.

Field CS, Ory SJ, Wahner HW, Herrmann RR, Judd HL, Riggs BL. Preventive effects of transdermal 17ß-estradiol on osteoporotic changes after surgical menopause: a two-year placebo-controlled trial. *Am J Obstet Gynecol*. 1993;168:114-121.

Gallagher JC, Kable WT, Goldgar D. Effect of progestin therapy on cortical and trabecular bone: comparison with estrogen. *Am J Med*. 1991;90:171-178.

Gambacciani M, Spinetti A, Taponeco F, Cappagli B, Piaggesi L, Fioretti P. Longitudinal evaluation of perimenopausal vertebral bone loss: effects of a low-dose oral contraceptive preparation on bone mineral density and metabolism. *Obstet Gynecol*. 1994;83: 392-396.

Gebbie A. Risks and benefits of estrogen plus progestin in healthy postmenopausal women. Principal results from the Women's Health Initiative #10; Investigators. *JAMA*. 2002;288:321-333.

Genant HK, Baylink DJ, Gallagher JC, Harris ST, Steiger P, Herber M. Effect of estrone sulfate on postmenopausal bone loss. *Obstet Gynecol*. 1990;76:579-584.

11

Genant HK, Lucas J, Weiss S, et al. Low-dose esterified estrogen therapy: effects on bone, plasma estradiol concentrations, endometrium, and lipid levels. Estratab/Osteoporosis Study Group. *Arch Intern Med.* 1997;157:2609-2615.

Hammar ML, Lindgren R, Berg GE, Möller CG, Niklasson MK. Effects of hormonal replacement therapy on the postural balance among postmenopausal women. *Obstet Gynecol.* 1996;88:955-960.

Holland EF, Chow JW, Studd JW, Leather AT, Chambers TJ. Histomorphometric changes in the skeleton of postmenopausal women with low bone mineral density treated with percutaneous estradiol implants. *Obstet Gynecol.* 1994;83:387-391.

Horsman A, Jones M, Francis R, Nordin C. The effect of estrogen dose on postmenopausal bone loss. *N Engl J Med.* 1983;309:1405-1407.

Kleerekoper M. Lessons from the skeleton: was the Women's Health Initiative (WHI) a primary prevention trial? *Osteoporos Int.* 2002;13:685-687.

Leelawattana R, Ziambaras K, Roodman-Weiss J, et al. The oxidative metabolism of estradiol conditions postmenopausal bone density and bone loss. *J Bone Miner Res.* 2000;15:2513-2520.

Lindsay R, Gallagher JC, Kleerekoper M, Pickar JH. Effect of lower doses of conjugated equine estrogens with and without medroxyprogesterone acetate on bone in early postmenopausal women. *JAMA.* 2002;287:2668-2676.

Lindsay R, Hart DM, Clark DM. The minimum effective dose of estrogen for prevention of postmenopausal bone loss. *Obstet Gynecol.* 1984;63:759-763.

Lindsay R, Hart DM, Forrest C, Baird C. Prevention of spinal osteoporosis in oophorectomised women. *Lancet.* 1980;2: 1151-1154.

Lindsay R, Hart DM, MacLean A, Clark AC, Kraszewski A, Garwood J. Bone response to termination of oestrogen treatment. *Lancet.* 1978;1:1325-1327.

Lindsay R, Tohme JF. Estrogen treatment of patients with established postmenopausal osteoporosis. *Obstet Gynecol.* 1990;76:290-295.

226

Lufkin EG, Wahner HW, O'Fallon WM, et al. Treatment of postmenopausal osteoporosis with transdermal estrogen. *Ann Intern Med*. 1992;117:1-9.

Marshall RW, Selby PL, Chilvers DC, Hodgkinson A. The effect of ethinyl oestradiol on calcium and bone metabolism in peri- and postmenopausal women. *Horm Metab Res*. 1984; 16:97-99.

Maxim P, Ettinger B, Spitalny GM. Fracture protection provided by long-term estrogen treatment. *Osteoporos Int*. 1995;5:23-29.

Moore M, Bracker M, Sartoris D, Saltman P, Strause L. Long-term estrogen replacement therapy in postmenopausal women sustains vertebral bone mineral density. *J Bone Miner Res*. 1990;5:659-664.

Munk-Jensen N, Pors Nielsen S, Obel EB, Bonne Eriksen P. Reversal of postmenopausal vertebral bone loss by oestrogen and progestogen: a double blind placebo controlled study. *Br Med J*. 1988;296:1150-1152.

NIH Consensus Development Panel on Osteoporosis Prevention, Diagnosis, and Therapy. Osteoporosis prevention, diagnosis, and therapy. *JAMA*. 2001;285:758-795.

Notelovitz M. Androgen effects on bone and muscle. *Fertil Steril*. 2002;77(suppl 4):S34-S41.

Notelovitz M. Estrogen therapy and osteoporosis: principles and practice. *Am J Med Sci*. 1997;313:2-12.

Notelovitz M. Osteoporosis: screening, prevention, and management. *Fertil Steril*. 1993;59:707-725.

Notelovitz M, John VA, Good WR. Effectiveness of Alora estradiol matrix transdermal delivery system in improving lumbar bone mineral density in healthy, postmenopausal women. *Menopause*. 2002;9:343-353.

Notelovitz M, Johnston M, Smith S, Kitchens C. Metabolic and hormonal effects of 25-mg and 50-mg 17ß-estradiol implants in surgically menopausal women. *Obstet Gynecol*. 1987;70:749-754.

Notelovitz M, Varner RE, Rebar RW, et al. Minimal endometrial proliferation over a two-year period in postmenopausal women taking 0.3 mg of unopposed esterified estrogens. *Menopause*. 1997;4:80-88.

Phillips KA, Glendon G, Knight JA. Putting the risk of breast cancer in perspective. *N Engl J Med.* 1999;340:141-144.

Prior JC. Progesterone as a bone-trophic hormone. *Endocr Rev.* 1990;11:386-398.

Rickard DJ, Waters KM, Ruesink TJ, et al. Estrogen receptor isoform-specific induction of progesterone receptors in human osteoblasts. *J Bone Miner Res.* 2002;17:580-592.

Salmen T, Heikkinen AM, Mahonen A, et al. The protective effect of hormone-replacement therapy on fracture risk is modulated by estrogen receptor alpha genotype in early postmenopausal women. *J Bone Miner Res.* 2000;15:2479-2486.

Scholes D, Lacroix AZ, Ott SM, Ichikawa LE, Barlow WE. Bone mineral density in women using depot medroxyprogesterone acetate for contraception. *Obstet Gynecol.* 1999;93:233-238.

Speroff L. The Heart and Estrogen/Progestin Replacement Study (HERS). *Maturitas.* 1998;31:9-14.

Speroff L. Postmenopausal hormone therapy and breast cancer. *Obstet Gynecol.* 1996;87(suppl 2):44S-54S.

Speroff L, Rowan J, Symons J, Genant H, Wilborn W. The comparative effect on bone density, endometrium, and lipids of continuous hormones as replacement therapy (CHART study). A randomized controlled trial. *JAMA.* 1996;276:1397-1403.

Trabal JF, Lenihan JP Jr, Melchione TE, et al. Low-dose unopposed estrogens: preliminary findings on the frequency and duration of vaginal bleeding in postmenopausal women receiving esterified estrogens over a two-year period. *Menopause.* 1997;4:130-138.

Verborgt O, Gibson GJ, Schaffler MB. Loss of osteocyte integrity in associaton with microdamage and bone remodeling after fatigue in vivo. *J Bone Miner Res.* 2000;15:60-67.

Villareal DT, Binder EF, Williams DB, Schechtman KB, Yarasheski KE, Kohrt WM. Bone mineral density response to estrogen replacement in frail elderly women: a randomized controlled trial. *JAMA.* 2001;286:815-820.

Weiss NS, Treggiari MM. Postmenopausal hormone use and skeletal fracture: does the size of the benefit decrease with increasing age? *Obstet Gynecol.* 2002;100;364-368.

12 Drug Therapy Alternatives to Hormone Therapy: Antiresorptives

Drug Classes

Based on the pathophysiology of the bone remodeling cycle, drugs used to prevent and/or treat osteoporosis fall into two main classes:

- *Antiresorptive agents*:
  - These drugs inhibit osteoclast activity and are especially useful in patients with rapid bone remodeling.
  - Most of the drugs in clinical practice today are in this category and include:
    - Estrogen
    - Bisphosphonates
    - Selective estrogen receptor modulators (SERMS)
    - Calcitonin.
- *Bone formation stimulants*:
  - Bone remodeling stimulants and bone formation–stimulating regimens increase bone formation more than bone resorption and result in sustained substantial increases in bone mass.
  - Sodium fluoride, androgens (possibly), and parathyroid hormone (PTH).

Anticipated Clinical Outcomes

As illustrated in Figure 12.1, the rate and degree of bone mineral density (BMD) change will vary ac-

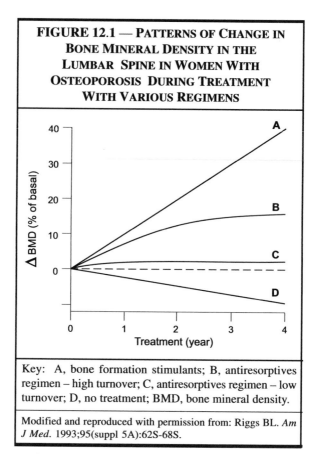

FIGURE 12.1 — PATTERNS OF CHANGE IN BONE MINERAL DENSITY IN THE LUMBAR SPINE IN WOMEN WITH OSTEOPOROSIS DURING TREATMENT WITH VARIOUS REGIMENS

Key: A, bone formation stimulants; B, antiresorptives regimen – high turnover; C, antiresorptives regimen – low turnover; D, no treatment; BMD, bone mineral density.

Modified and reproduced with permission from: Riggs BL. *Am J Med.* 1993;95(suppl 5A):62S-68S.

cording to the underlying etiology of the patient's osteopenia/osteoporosis and the class of drug used:

- With antiresorptive therapy, an 8% to 20% gain in BMD can be anticipated if the bone turnover rate is high. A plateau in gain will be reached after 2 to 3 years.
- In patients with low or normal bone-turnover rates, the bone mass will be stabilized or increase more modestly. However, this does not necessarily indicate inferior protection against fracture.

- Use of bone formation–stimulating drugs such as sodium fluoride can result in a linear 10%/year increase in BMD for at least 4 years. Similar results have now been recorded for PTH.

Estrogen is discussed in detail in Chapter 11, *Postmenopausal Hormone Therapy*. The other anti-resorptive agents are bisphosphonates, SERMS, and calcitonin.

Bisphosphonates

■ Pharmacology

Bisphosphonates are synthetic compounds that have a nonhydrolyzable P-C-P bond that adheres strongly to hydroxyapatite crystals of bone. There are two side chains:
- One binds to bone mineral
- One determines potency (nitrogen molecule).

The first generation of bisphosphonates are non-amino compounds:
- Clondronate
- Etidronate
- Pamidronate.

The second generation or aminobisphosphonates include:
- Alendronate
- Risedronate.

Third generation bisphosphonates under development include:
- Ibandronate
- Zoledronic acid.

Potency of the drugs depends on the length and structure of the side chain (Figure 12.2).

12

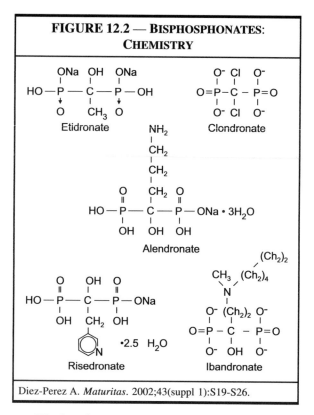

FIGURE 12.2 — BISPHOSPHONATES: CHEMISTRY

Etidronate

Clondronate

Alendronate

Risedronate

Ibandronate

Diez-Perez A. *Maturitas*. 2002;43(suppl 1):S19-S26.

Bisphosphonates accumulate in the acid environment between the bone and osteoclasts. They also:

- Suppress bone resorption by interfering with activation of osteoclasts
- Greatly slow bone turnover, thus creating a smaller "remodeling space."

Newer research aimed at understanding how the bisphosphonates protect bone has established the following pathways:

- Decrease in the differentiation and recruitment of osteoclast precursor cells from the common hematopoietic stem cell. This decreases the number of mature active osteoclasts.

- Inhibition of integrins. The integrins are the main component of the seal that attaches the osteoclast to the bone surface. The seal facilitates the acid milieu below the osteoclast, which results in "old bone" being resorbed.
- Activation of the caspase system that results in the inhibition of the mevalonate pathway (involved in cholesterol production and statin activity) and the blocking of proteins responsible for the cytoskeletal organization of the osteoclast and for osteoclast cell proliferation and apoptosis.
- As noted previously, osteoblasts are responsible for the early activation and recruitment of osteoclast percursors, via the so-called RANK-RANKL system. This is inhibited by the aminobisphosphonates, which in addition, stimulate osteoblast number and function.
- Aminobisphosphonates prevent the apoptosis of osteocytes.

Oral absorption is ± 1% to 3% of the dose and is decreased by food or calcium. Calcium binds the drug in the gut. Bisphosphonates are released slowly from the skeleton and adhesion of the bisphosphonates to the bone is very long and may be a lifetime. About 30% to 50% of the absorbed dose adheres to the active bone surfaces and the rest is excreted in urine.

12

■ Drugs Available
Alendronate
Alendronate (Fosamax) was the first bisphosphonate used in clinical practice and, unlike etidronate, permits effective inhibition of osteoclast-mediated bone resorption at doses that do not impair bone min-

eralization. Thus the newer, more potent agent may be taken daily.

A significant reduction in hip, wrist, and vertebral fractures has now been found by investigators in the 36- to 48-month Fracture Interventional Trial (FIT), a randomized, double-blind, placebo-controlled study of alendronate in women with low femoral neck bone mass density without vertebral fracture and in a cohort of women with existing vertebral fracture.

The results showed the following reductions in the relative risk (RR) of fracture:

- 53% for the hip (RR 0.47, 0.26-0.79)
- 48% radiographic vertebral fracture (RR 0.52, 0.42-0.66)
- 45% in clinical vertebral fractures (RR 0.55; 0.36-0.82).

Reductions in the risk of clinical fractures were statistically significant by 12 months into the trial. The dosage in this trial was 5 mg daily for 2 years, followed by 10 mg for the following year.

Another placebo-controlled study of postmenopausal women with low BMD showed a 47% reduction in the risk of nonvertebral fractures after 1 year of 10 mg alendronate daily. Alendronate, 5 mg and 10 mg daily, is FDA approved for both the prevention and treatment of osteoporosis. In order to improve compliance with therapy, a study comparing 70 mg alendronate in one weekly dose vs 10 mg daily for one week showed equal efficacy and safety for both regimens. Some researchers have found that stoppage of alendronate after prolonged use results in a loss of bone equivalent to that found in the early menopause. Alendronate (10 mg/day) was also effective in increasing the BMD of elderly women (65 years and older) in long-term care facilities.

It has not as yet been established whether it is safe to administer alendronate (or other bisphosphonates) after recent fracture. Fracture incidence is reduced after alendronate, and bone remodeling and turnover are decreased to the degree found in premenopausal women. Also, studies with the various bisphosphonates have all shown a positive effect on the mechanical characteristics of normal bone. As long as inhibition of mineralization is avoided, it would appear that bisphosphonates in the doses usually prescribed for osteoporosis prevention/treatment are safe to use in subjects who have recently experienced fracture—but there are no human data to support (or refute) this conclusion. Decisions will have to be based on the circumstances of the individual case.

In a 2-year study comparing 5 mg alendronate and combination hormone therapy (HT) (0.625 mg conjugated equine estrogen [CEE] and 5 mg of medroxyprogesterone acetate [MPA]), equivalent increases in the BMD of the spine and hip were noted. The respective increase in lumbar BMD was 3.5% and 4.0%; the total hip enhancement was almost identical: 1.83% and 1.85%. Women in the placebo group lost 1.78% of total lumbar BMD and 1.42% from the total hip. Drug-related side effects and discontinuation of the study because of adverse experiences are summarized in Figure 12.3. Thus 5 mg alendronate daily is an effective agent in preventing bone loss in recently postmenopausal women. Because of its low prevalence of side effects, 5 mg alendronate daily is especially useful in women who:

- Have contraindications for HT
- Have clinically significant side effects (such as mastalgia)
- Will not take HT because of their fear of breast cancer and/or resumption of menstruation.

A recent study has shown that combining estrogen and alendronate therapy results in a modest—but significantly greater—increase in BMD compared

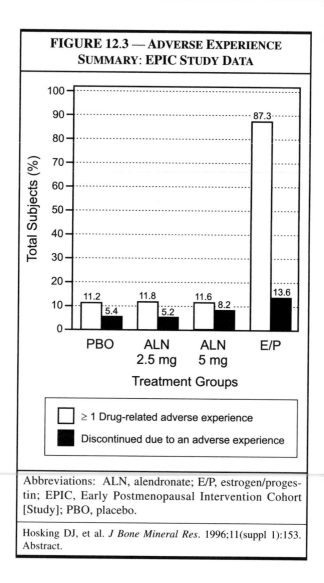

FIGURE 12.3 — ADVERSE EXPERIENCE SUMMARY: EPIC STUDY DATA

Abbreviations: ALN, alendronate; E/P, estrogen/progestin; EPIC, Early Postmenopausal Intervention Cohort [Study]; PBO, placebo.

Hosking DJ, et al. *J Bone Mineral Res.* 1996;11(suppl 1):153. Abstract.

with either estrogen or alendronate-alone therapy. Adding 5 mg alendronate to women on estrogen therapy (ET) for climacteric complaints achieved an increase in BMD equivalent to that achieved by 10 mg alendronate daily. Alendronate (5 mg and 10 mg daily doses) has been found to be effective in the treatment of glucocorticoid-induced osteoporosis.

Side Effects

Although side effects were generally minimal (abdominal and musculoskeletal pain, nausea, dyspepsia, constipation, diarrhea, and, rarely rash), about 3% of patients in one study developed esophageal ulcers. Of the 211 esophageal reactions to alendronic acid reported worldwide, 36 were serious; in about half the reported cases, the drug had not been taken in accordance with the prescribing information (with inadequate amount of water or patient did not remain upright for 30 minutes or more). A more recent study of 6432 men and women found that although there was a threefold increase in risk for gastrointestinal (GI) problems, much of this association was due to comorbid conditions and other factors. Alendronate 70 mg once weekly was not associated with any increase in endoscopic lesions in the upper GI tract relative to placebo.

Regimen

An alendronate regimen should include:
- 5 or 10 mg/day, with 6 to 8 oz water, on arising, at least one half hour before breakfast. Patient should remain sitting up or erect for at least 30 minutes to 1 hour
- Calcium supplements and antacids interfere with absorption of alendronate; thus they should be taken at least one half hour later

- No dosage adjustment is necessary for the elderly or for patients with mild-to-moderate renal insufficiency
- Same regimen if alendronate is taken in a single 70-mg dose.

Seven years of therapy with alendronate is safe. There may, however, be no additional benefit after 5 years based on changes in BMD and bone markers.

Risedronate

Risedronate (Actonel) is a second-generation aminobisphosphonate approved for the prevention and treatment of postmenopausal osteoporosis. It is administered orally in a dose of one 5-mg tablet daily or one 35-mg tablet taken once weekly. Risedronate has been studied in a number of randomized controlled trials and in at least seven clinical trials. Based on these trials, risedronate 5 mg daily has been shown to significantly increase the BMD of the spine and hip in women with established osteoporosis within and beyond 5 years of menopause. Increases in BMD are measurable within 6 months, and possibly as early as 3 months, of starting treatment.

Risedronate significantly reduced the cumulative incidence of new vertebral fractures in patients by 41% over 3 years and by 65% after the first year in women with prevalent fractures (Figure 12.4). The comparable reduction in vertebral fractures in a large multinational study was 49% after 3 years of treatment and 61% within the first year following the initiation of the trial.

Nonvertebral fractures are reduced by 30% to 40%. In elderly women (aged 70 to 79 years) with BMD-defined osteoporosis, hip fracture incidence was reduced by 40%, and by 60% in those women with prevalent vertebral fractures after 3 years of risedronate treatment (Figure 12.5). There was no significant reduction in hip fractures in women older than 80 years and who were admitted into the trial on the basis of clinical risk factors for falls, but not necessarily with BMD-diagnosed osteoporosis.

Risedronate normalizes the biochemical markers of bone modeling. Bone formed during risedronate treatment is histologically normal. Animal studies have demonstrated that risedronate preserves the trabecular architecture in the vertebrae of ovariectomized pigs.

Risedronate prevents vertebral bone loss in patients initiating or continuing long-term corticosteroid therapy. This was associated with a 70% reduction in vertebral fracture risk. In addition, risedronate preserves BMD in women with breast cancer who have chemotherapy-induced menopause.

One year of estrogen-alone therapy (CEE 0.625 mg daily) or combined with 5 mg risedronate daily has a similar favorable effect on the spine BMD (ET alone 4.6% >; ET plus risedronate 5.2% >), femoral neck (1.8% and 2.7%, respectively), and on the distal and midshaft areas of the radius.

Side Effects

Some of the gastric side effects associated with bisphosphonate therapy are thought to be due to their interference with the surface hydrophobic phospholipid barrier of gastric tissue. This is said to be more common in patients treated with primary vs second-generation bisphosphonates, and is accounted for by structural differences in the two types of nitrogen-containing drugs.

A recent head-to-head study compared the incidence of both gastric ulcers of esophageal and GI injury following 5 mg risedronate or 10 mg alendronate. Subjects underwent endoscopy at baseline and after 2 weeks of treatment. The result: only 4.1% in the risedronate group compared with 13.2% in the

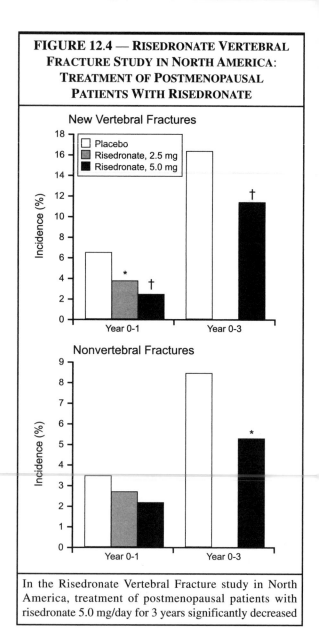

FIGURE 12.4 — RISEDRONATE VERTEBRAL FRACTURE STUDY IN NORTH AMERICA: TREATMENT OF POSTMENOPAUSAL PATIENTS WITH RISEDRONATE

New Vertebral Fractures

Placebo
Risedronate, 2.5 mg
Risedronate, 5.0 mg

Nonvertebral Fractures

In the Risedronate Vertebral Fracture study in North America, treatment of postmenopausal patients with risedronate 5.0 mg/day for 3 years significantly decreased the incidence of new vertebral fractures *(top)* and combined incidence of new vertebral fractures or nonvertebral fractures *(bottom)*. The risedronate 2.5 mg/day group was discontinued before the end of the study.

* *P* <0.05.
† *P* <0.05 vs placebo.

Harris ST, et al. *JAMA*. 1999;282:1344-1352.

FIGURE 12.5 — RISEDRONATE VS PLACEBO: KAPLAN-MEIER ESTIMATES OF THE INCIDENCE OF HIP FRACTURE

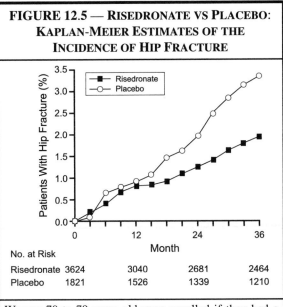

No. at Risk			
Risedronate	3624	3040	2681	2464
Placebo	1821	1526	1339	1210

Women 70 to 79 years old were enrolled if they had a low bone mineral density at the femoral neck (T-score, lower than -4 or lower than -3 with at least one nonskeletal risk factor for hip fracture).

McClung MR, et al. *N Engl J Med*. 2001;344:333-340.

alendronate group were observed to have developed gastric ulcers.

Dosing

As with other bisphosphonates, the intestinal absorption of risedronate is low and averages 0.63% in healthy volunteers. The absorption of risedronate is decreased by 55% if the medication is taken <30 minutes before breakfast or 2 hours after dinner. Consequently, risedronate is recommended to be taken at least 30 minutes before the first food or drink of the day (except water), without lying down for 30 minutes afterward. The preliminary results of a study comparing risedronate 5 mg daily, 35 mg weekly, or 50 mg weekly showed equivalent results in lumbar BMD improvement after 1 year of therapy: 4.0%, 3.94%, and 4.25%, respectively. Changes in hip BMD were also similar in all three groups and there was no difference among the three groups in tolerability.

■ Third-Generation Bisphosphonates

A third generation of bisphosphonates is presently in clinical trial. These drugs are even more potent and have the advantage of being able to be given by injection or orally.

Ibandronate

This bisphosphonate has twice the potency of risedronate and ten times the potency of alendronate. Because of the high affinity of bisphosphonates to bone and the prolonged effect on bone after being absorbed onto the bone surface, the intermittent use of ibandronate has been evaluated. The clinical trials have involved both 3 monthly 1-mg IV injections and, more recently, intermittent oral therapy. The latter regimen involved 20 mg ibandronate every other day for 24 days, followed by 9 weeks of no therapy. Anticipated increases in BMD in the spine (5.4%) and the hip (3.4%) were recorded, with a decrease in the relevant biochemical markers of bone turnover. It should be noted, however, that although the IV ibandronate therapy increased BMD of the spine (4% higher than that of the placebo group), this regimen only decreased spinal fractures by a modest 26%.

Zoledronic Acid

Zoledronic acid (ZA) is the most potent bisphosphonate studied to date. In a phase 2 clinical trial, postmenopausal women who were ≥ 5 years postmenopause and who had a BMD with a T-score ≥ -2, were treated with either IV placebo, 0.25 mg, 0.5 mg, or 1 mg ZA at 3 monthly intervals, 6 monthly doses 2 mg ZA, or an annual IV dose of 40 mg ZA. All doses resulted in a similar increase in spinal BMD (5%) compared with placebo and even with the once-a-year injection, a 52% decrease in serum C-telopeptide and a 65% decrease in urinary N-telopeptide excretion. There were, however, more treatment-related side effects (musculoskeletal pain, nausea, or fever) in the ZA-treated women (45% to 67%) compared with the placebo group (27%).

Neither ibandronate nor ZA is presently available for clinical use.

■ Other Bisphosphonates

A number of other bisphosphonates have been developed and are used for the treatment of malignant diseases of bone and Paget's disease of bone. These include:

- Clondronate
- Tiludronate
- Pamidronate
- Etidronate.

The latter is prescribed in Europe for the treatment of osteoporosis but is not approved by the Food and Drug Administration (FDA) for this indication in the United States.

In the author's opinion, the off-label use of etidronate (Didronel) provides a viable option for women with contraindications or intolerance to HT and the approved bisphosphonates. Etidronate needs to be prescribed cyclically as follows:

- 400 mg daily for 2 weeks
- Taken on an empty stomach or mid afternoon (ie, between lunch and dinner)
- No calcium supplements for the 2 weeks of treatment
- Dosage is repeated every 3 months.

The results of a 4-year study comparing intermittent cyclic etidronate (ICE) alone, HT alone (CEE 0.625 mg daily and norgestrel 150 mcg for 12 days per month); combination ICE and HT therapy, or calcium and vitamin D are summarized in Figure 12.6. BMD increased most in the combination therapy group in both the spine (10.4%) and in the hip (7.0%) at the end of 4 years. The etidronate-alone results for the spine 7.3%) and hip (0.9%) and for the HT-alone group (spine 7.0%; hip 4.8%) were significantly less than those recorded for the combination therapy group.

Selective Estrogen Receptor Modulators

■ Raloxifene (Evista)
Systemic Effects

Raloxifene is a selective estrogen-receptor modulator. It binds to estrogen receptors (ER) (primarily ERα) in bone, breast, and uterine cells but acts as an estrogen antagonist in breast and uterus and an agonist in bone and the cardiovascular system. Studies

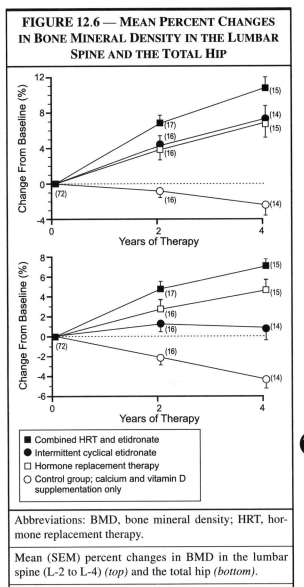

FIGURE 12.6 — MEAN PERCENT CHANGES IN BONE MINERAL DENSITY IN THE LUMBAR SPINE AND THE TOTAL HIP

- ■ Combined HRT and etidronate
- ● Intermittent cyclical etidronate
- □ Hormone replacement therapy
- ○ Control group; calcium and vitamin D supplementation only

Abbreviations: BMD, bone mineral density; HRT, hormone replacement therapy.

Mean (SEM) percent changes in BMD in the lumbar spine (L-2 to L-4) *(top)* and the total hip *(bottom)*.

Wimalawansa SJ. *Am J Med*. 1998;104:219-226.

12

have shown a 60% to 70% reduction in breast cancer risk with use of raloxifene, however, it is not FDA approved for this indication.

Beneficial effects of raloxifene on serum lipids are about half as effective as those of conjugated estrogens 0.625 mg but without uterine-stimulating effects. Animal studies suggest that the lipid-lowering effect of raloxifene compared with conjugated estrogen is not associated with a reduction in coronary artery atherosclerosis. Clinical studies have not demonstrated a negative cardiovascular effect in women.

There is some concern regarding the potential antiestrogen central nervous system effect of raloxifene:

- Hot flash symptoms are provoked in 28.7% of previously asymptomatic menopausal women on a 60-mg once-daily dose of raloxifene vs 3.1% of women on continuous combined HT (0.625 mg CEE plus 2.5 mg MPA)
- A recent study showed no cognitive impairment in postmenopausal women compared with placebo-treated controls, but also no improvement (although in two studies, raloxifene-treated women did better than controls in two tests of verbal memory and attention)
- A preliminary study shows that raloxifene may impair balance.

Raloxifene may be the treatment of choice for women who:

- Are at high risk for breast cancer
- Have modest degrees of osteopenia
- Have hypertriglyceridemia.

Bone

In early postmenopausal women, raloxifene prevents postmenopausal bone loss in all skeletal sites (2.7% at the lumbar spine and 2.4% at the femoral neck

246

after 3 years of 60 mg raloxifene daily), but to a lesser degree than that following ET and HT.

It reduces bone markers of bone turnover to premenopausal levels. This probably results from the blocking of cytokines that promote osteoclast differentiations.

A 3-year trial (Multiple Outcomes of Raloxifene Evaluation [MORE]) resulted in a 30% reduction of vertebral fractures in women with prevalent fractures and a 50% reduction of spinal fractures in women without prevalent fractures. No reduction in nonvertebral fractures was noted. The paradox between the modest increase in lumbar BMD but robust decrease in the incidence of vertebral fracture has been attributed to raloxifene's ability to inhibit perforation of the trabecular plates, thereby maintaining the structural integrity (and strength) of the microarchitecture of cancellous bone. This may be a mechanism of action common to all antiresorptive agents. Only doses of antiresorptive drugs greater than the equivalent 60-mg dose of raloxifene will produce larger increases in BMD. The latter will probably require treatment with bone formation–stimulating therapies PTH (see Chapter 13).

Although rare, thromboembolic disease (venous thrombosis [RR 1.78] and pulmonary embolism [RR 2.76]) is increased. The RR is similar to that seen with HT.

12

Dosage

Raloxifene is approved for the prevention of osteoporosis. The daily dose is 60 mg.

■ **Tamoxifen**

Tamoxifen, the first identified SERM, is also an estrogen antagonist in breast tissue, with partial agonism in bone. However, tamoxifen also has estrogen agonist activity in the endometrium (unlike raloxifene) and is associated with rare but aggressive endometrial cancer. This precludes its use in healthy postmenopausal women.

■ Tibolone (Livial)

Tibolone is a synthetic steroid described as a tissue-specific drug that acts through its metabolites on estrogen, progesterone, and androgen receptors. Tibolone prevents bone loss in perimenopausal and late postmenopausal women. No fracture data are available. Tibolone has an excellent clinical profile, such as:

- Reducing hot flashes and symptoms of urogenital atrophy
- Inhibiting the endometrium and has a good bleeding profile
- Lowering elevated levels of cholesterol, triglycerides, and low-density lipoprotein (LDL) cholesterol.

Adverse side effects include:

- Slight increase in venous thromboembolism comparable to that associated with HT
- Approximately 30% decrease in high-density lipoprotein (HDL) cholesterol. This has, however, been explained by an increase in the efficiency of the HDL–reverse cholesterol transport system and, in animal studies, has not been associated with an increase in atherogenic disease.

Daily dose is 2.5 mg. Lower doses (1.25 mg) maybe equally effective in some women. Tibolone is used widely in Europe but has not as yet been FDA approved for use in the United States.

Calcitonin

Calcitonin is a polypeptide hormone produced by the parafollicular C cells of the thyroid.

Calcitonin has antiosteoclastic activity:

- Osteoclasts have receptors that bind calcitonin
- Calcitonin inhibits osteoclasts by:
  - Interfering with osteoclast brush borders
  - Inhibiting cytoplasmic motility
  - Decreasing the rate of osteoclast formation.

■ Types of Preparations Available

In clinical practice, the most commonly used calcitonin is derived from salmon. Other preparations are derived from human, pig, and an analog of eel calcitonin.

Salmon calcitonin (SCT) is administered either:

- Parenterally, by:
  - Intramuscular (IM) injection
  - Subcutaneous (SC) injection
- Intranasally
- More recently, an oral formulation of SCT is under development.

Available SCT products are listed in Table 12.1.

Parenteral SCT is indicated for Paget's disease, hypercalcemia, and postmenopausal osteoporosis. Some clinically relevant facts include:

- Acts essentially identical to mammalian calcitonins, but its potency and duration of action are greater.
- The majority of randomized, placebo-controlled studies demonstrate greater bone density in calcitonin-treated patients as early as 3 months after initiation of therapy, with persistence for up to 3 years.
- Effective analgesic therapy for pain of acute and chronic osteoporotic vertebral fractures.
- Evidence of calcitonin's efficacy in fracture prevention is limited. In a randomized placebo-controlled study (PROOF study) in postmenopausal women with osteoporosis, 200 IU intra-

12

TABLE 12.1 — SALMON CALCITONIN PREPARATIONS

Brand Name	How Supplied	Manufacturer
Parenteral		
Miacalcin Injection Subcutaneously or intramuscularly	2-mL multiple-dose vials (200 IU/mL)	Novartis
Intranasal		
Miacalcin Nasal Spray	2-mL bottles with pump (200 IU per activation, 0.09 mL/spray)	Novartis

nasal SCT reduced the rate of vertebral fractures by 30% in comparison with placebo. No significant reduction in peripheral fractures were noted. There was also no consistent effect on bone markers and BMD. Doses of 100 and 400 IU had no effect.

- Side effects, inconvenient rather than serious, including anorexia, nausea, vomiting, metallic taste, diarrhea, flushing, rash, and pruritus.

Intranasal SCT, which is indicated for the treatment of osteoporosis in women who are >5 years postmenopause with low bone mass, has the following characteristics:

- Clinical and biologic effects similar to those of the IM version
- Mean bioavailability of the nasal spray approximately 3% of that of injectable calcitonin in normal subjects
- Production of significant increases in lumbar vertebral BMD as early as 6 months, with persistence up to 2 years. Although the increase in BMD is relatively modest compared with that of the other antiresorptive drugs, long-term calcitonin therapy has been associated with a 30% to 35% reduction in fractures
- No effects on cortical bone of forearm or hip demonstrated
- Tolerance better than with the parenteral route of administration
- Rhinitis, epistaxis, and sinusitis have occurred in 12%, 3.5%, and 2.3% of patients, respectively.

Oral SCT, which relies on a specialized amino acid derivative as an intestinal carrier, has been developed and produces all the biologic effects of calcitonin. The tolerability of the preparation is good, but

12

because the intestinal absorption of peptides is limited, 1000 µg is required by the oral route to reproduce the concentrations and effects of an intravenous (IV) infusion of 10 µg. The drug is in phase 1 trials.

■ Clinical Practice

Salmon calcitonin injections serve two main purposes:

- Inhibition of bone loss; especially in patients with increased calcium-to-creatinine ratios (high turnover bone loss) and increased collagen cross-link excretion.
- Analgesia: Pain relief in 66% of patients with Paget's disease who are treated with parenteral calcitonin; pain relief is due to:
  - An increase in circulating β-endorphin
  - Direct effect on pain threshold centers in the central nervous system.

Parenteral SCT is, therefore, useful in postfracture situations. Added benefits include:

- Reduction in the duration of bed confinement
- Reduction in the number of concomitant analgesics.

Intranasal SCT is a substitute for the IM or SC forms only for patients with established osteoporosis of at least 5 years' duration, not for those in early menopause.

■ Regimens

Calcitonin regimens vary with the clinical situation and cost of drug therapy. Suggested regimens are:

- *Parenteral form*:
  - Postfracture: 100 IU/day SC for 6 to 8 weeks (the analgesic dose is thought to be 100 IU/day)
  - 100 IU 3 times a week for the next 6 months

- Maintenance: 50 IU 3 times a week
- Monitor the progress with monthly urinary calcium-to-creatinine ratios and urinary collagen cross-link excretion
- Depending on the initial bone density, dual-energy x-ray absorptiometry (DEXA) analysis should be repeated every 6 to 12 months.
- *Nasal spray*:
  - Screw-on pump, once primed, delivers a metered dose of 0.09 mL/spray
  - Dose is one spray (200 IU) per day, alternating nostrils daily
  - Drug effect may be monitored by periodic measurements of lumbar vertebral bone mass. The nasal spray's effects on biochemical markers of bone turnovers have not been consistently demonstrated and should not be used as the sole markers of clinical response
  - Periodic nasal examinations are recommended.

■ Special Conditions Suited to Calcitonin Therapy

Although not FDA approved, parenteral calcitonin has also been found to be potentially useful in steroid-induced osteoporosis. *Precautions include*:

- High doses of calcitonin (>200 IU/day) in the absence of calcium supplementation can induce secondary hyperparathyroidism. Ensure that the patient has a calcium supplement/intake of at least 1500 g/day.
- Subclinical forms of vitamin D deficiency (25-hydroxyvitamin D values <10 ng/mL) will blunt the skeletal response to calcitonin.

■ Long-term Compliance

- Patients with no clinical symptoms or signs of osteoporosis are reluctant to continue therapy.

- Development of antibodies and down-regulation of calcitonin receptors limit the drug's clinical usefulness after 2 or more years of therapy. Since down-regulation is more likely, treatment should be stopped after 2 to 3 years for 6 months and then reinitiated. Biochemical parameters and bone density should be monitored during this period.

Other Drugs

■ Statins

A series of studies have suggested that the statin class of drugs (HMG-CoA reductase inhibitors) are associated with a reduction in fracture risk. There is a linkage between the pharmacologic action of these lipid-lowering drugs and the pathogenesis of osteoporosis.

Mevalonic acid is a precursor of cholesterol and also of a series of proteins, such as geranylgeranyl pyrophosphate (GGP), which control osteoclast-mediated bone resorption. The aminobisphosphonates exert their pharmacologic antiresorptive action (in part) by inhibiting the formation of GGP.

Of the seven studies published to date, most of which are observational, three confirmed the relationship between statin use and a reduction in fracture risk, and four did not show a statistically significant protective effect. The data refer only to hip fracture and many of the studies are confounded by factors such as existing obesity, physical activity, and other nutritional variables. Until prospective trials evaluating osteoporosis-related fracture end points are available, it is best to limit the use of statins to patients with hyperlipidemia, and drugs with proven antifracture efficacy to the treatment of osteopenia and osteoporosis.

A number of other treatments are used in some countries for the treatment of osteoporosis and include the following:

- Vitamin D_3 analogs (calcitriol):
  - Vitamin D decreases bone resorption secondary to an increase in calcium absorption
  - A decrease in calcium absorption (especially in the elderly) may be due to an impairment in hydroxylation of 25-hydroxyvitamin D to $1,25\text{-}(OH)_2D_3$, the active metabolite needed for calcium absorption
  - Vitamin D may also be an indirect stimulator of bone resorption via receptor-mediated activity on osteoblasts, and it has the ability to enhance the differentiation of preosteoclasts to osteoclasts
  - Calcitriol improves and may normalize impaired calcitonin secretion in mildly vitamin D–deficient elderly subjects
  - 1-α-hydroxyanalogs of vitamin D_3 have been synthesized ($1\text{-}(OH)D_3$-alphacalcidiol) but are very potent and may result in hypercalcemia
  - If calcitriol is to be used, the following precautions are recommended:
    - Restrict dietary calcium to 700 to 800 mg/day
    - Monitor urinary calcium; keep levels <300 mg/day
    - Increase daily water intake
- Ipriflavone
- Vitamin K
- Strontium ranelaze
- Growth hormone
- Thiazide diuretics.

12

The reader is referred to the literature for more detailed information.

Choosing an Antiresorptive Agent

The availability of many drugs for the prevention and/or treatment of osteoporosis has increased the complexity of clinical decision making for both the physician and the patient.

The new gold standard for evaluating the efficacy of long-term therapy is the randomized clinical trial (RCT) with clinical end points (fracture) as the determining end point rather than the previously relied upon surrogate markers (BMD and biochemical bone markers).

Tables 12.2 and 12.3 summarize the meta-analysis of some of the more commonly used therapies for the treatment of postmenopausal osteoporosis.

■ Clinical Interpretation

The data summarized in Tables 12.2 and 12.3 represent the results of studies performed in selected groups of individuals who had to meet special protocol criteria. Furthermore, they were randomized into treatment groups for the duration of study, absent severe adverse events, without reference to their interim clinical response. This is appropriate for an RCT but is not the standard that should be applied to the clinical care of individuals. Postmenopausal osteoporosis may present with the same diagnostic criteria (reduced BMD and fragility fractures), but the etiology is often different. Further, the patient may have additional medical needs that would influence a given therapy. Factors that should be considered on an individual basis and adjusted over time according to the patient's treatment response include:

- Bone health evaluation as assessed by:
  - BMD: degree of bone loss

TABLE 12.2 — LUMBAR SPINE

Intervention	Effect on BMD (%)	Fracture Reduction RR (%)
Calcium	1.66	0.77 (23)
Vitamin D	0.41	0.63 (37)
Alendronate (5 mg)	5.81	0.52 (48)
Alendronate (10-40 mg)	7.48	—
Risedronate (5 mg)	4.54	0.64 (36)
Etidronate (400 mg)	4.06	0.63 (37)
Calcitonin (250-2800 IU/wk)	3.74	0.79 (21)
Raloxifene (60 mg)	2.51	0.60 (40)
Hormone therapy	6.76	0.60 (34)

Abbreviations: BMD, bone mineral density; RR, relative risk.

Adapted from: Cranney A, et al. *Endocr Rev.* 2002;23:570-578.

12

TABLE 12.3 — HIP

Intervention	Effect on BMD (%)	Nonvertebral Fracture Reduction* RR (%)
Calcium	1.64	0.86 (14)
Vitamin D	1.00	0.77 (23)
Alendronate (5 mg)	3.37	0.87 (13)
Alendronate (10-40 mg)	4.24	0.51 (49)
Risedronate (5 mg)	2.73	0.73 (27)
Etidronate (400 mg)	2.35	0.99 (1)
Calcitonin (350-800 IU/wk)	3.80	0.80 (20)
Raloxifene (60 mg)	2.11	0.91 (9)
Hormone therapy	4.12	0.87 (13)

Abbreviations: BMD, bone mineral density; RR, relative risk.

* Although this table refers to the magnitude in reduction of nonvertebral fractures, the consistency of results across fractures is such that clinicians should apply the pooled RR reductions for nonvertebral fractures with hip fractures.

Adapted from: Cranney A, et al. *Endocr Rev.* 2002;23:570-578.

- Bone markers: low vs high turnover; osteopenia/osteoporosis
- X-ray: prevalent spinal fractures
- Clinical history and physical examination
  - Mammogram
  - Gynecologic examination
  - Musculoskeletal examination
  - Liver/renal function tests
  - Lipid profile
  - Secondary factors, eg, thyroid profile
- Drug history (allergies and/or intolerance to relevant drugs).

Based on the above, plus a consideration of the efficacy of the drugs listed in Tables 12.2 and 12.3, an appropriate choice can be made for a given individual at a specific point in time. Close observation and regular monitoring will ensure optimum care and results.

SUGGESTED READING

Alendronate

Adami S, Baroni MC, Broggini M, et al. Treatment of postmenopausal osteoporosis with continuous daily oral alendronate in comparison with either placebo or intranasal salmon calcitonin. *Osteoporos Int.* 1993;3(suppl 3):S21-S27.

Black DM, Cummings SR, Karpf DB, et al. Randomised trial of effect of alendronate on risk of fracture in women with existing vertebral fractures. Fracture Intervention Trial Research Group. *Lancet.* 1996;348:1535-1541.

Black DM, Reiss TF, Nevitt MC, Cauley J, Karpf D, Cummings SR. Design of the Fracture Intervention Trial. *Osteoporos Int.* 1993;3(suppl 3):S29-S39.

Black DM, Thompson DE, Bauer DC, et al. Fracture risk reduction with alendronate in women with osteoporosis: The Fracture Intervention Trial. FIT Research Group. *J Clin Endocrinol Metab.* 2000;85:4118-4124.

12

Chesnut CH III, Harris ST. Short-term effect of alendronate on bone mass and bone remodeling in postmenopausal women. *Osteoporos Int.* 1993;3(suppl 3):S17-S19.

Chesnut CH III, McClung MR, Ensrud KE, et al. Alendronate treatment of the postmenopausal osteoporotic woman: effect of multiple dosages on bone mass and bone remodeling. *Am J Med.* 1995;99:144-152.

Donahue JG, Chan KA, Andrade SE, et al. Gastric and duodenal safety of daily alendronate. *Arch Intern Med.* 2002;162:936-942.

Gertz BJ, Holland SD, Kline WF, Matuszewski BK, Porras AG. Clinical pharmacology of alendronate sodium. *Osteoporos Int.* 1993;3(suppl 3):S13-S16.

Greenspan SL, Bone G 3rd, Schnitzer TJ, et al, for the Alendronate Once-Weekly Study Group. Two-year results of once-weekly administration of alendronate 70 mg for the treatment of postmenopausal osteoporosis. *J Bone Miner Res.* 2002;17:1988-1996.

Greenspan SL, Schneider DL, McClung MR, et al. Alendronate improves bone mineral density in elderly women with osteoporosis residing in long-term care facilities. A randomized, double-blind, placebo-controlled trial. *Ann Intern Med.* 2002;136:742-746.

Hosking DJ, McClung MR, Ravn P, et al. Alendronate in the prevention of osteoporosis: EPIC Study two-year results. *J Bone Miner Res.* 1996;11(suppl 1):153. Abstract.

Lanza FL, Hunt RH, Thomson AB, Provenza JM, Blank MA. Endoscopic comparison of esophageal and gastroduodenal effects of risedronate and alendronate in postmenopausal women. *Gastroenterology.* 2000;119:631-638.

Lanza FL, Sahba B, Schwartz H, et al. The upper GI safety and tolerability of oral alendronate at a dose of 70 milligrams once weekly: a placebo-controlled endoscopy study. *Am J Gastroenterology.* 2002;97:58-64.

Liberman UA, Weiss SR, Bröll J, et al. Effect of oral alendronate on bone mineral density and the incidence of fractures in post-menopausal osteoporosis. The Alendronate Phase III Osteoporosis Treatment Study Group. *N Engl J Med.* 1995;333:1437-1443.

Palomba S, Orio F, Colao A, et al. Effect of estrogen replacement plus low-dose alendronate treatment on bone density in surgically postmenopausal women with osteoporosis. *J Clin Endocrinol Metab.* 2002;87:1502-1508.

Ravn P, Weiss SR, Rodriguez-Portales JA, et al. Alendronate in early postmenopausal women: effects on bone mass during long-term treatment and after withdrawal. Alendronate Osteoporosis Prevention Study Group. *J Clin Endocrinol Metab.* 2000;85: 1492-1497.

Rodan GA, Seedor JG, Balena R. Preclinical pharmacology of alendronate. *Osteoporos Int.* 1993;3(suppl 3):S7-S12.

Saag KG, Emkey R, Schnitzer TJ, et al. Alendronate for the prevention and treatment of glucocorticoid-induced osteoporosis. Glucocorticoid-Induced Osteoporosis Intervention Study Group. *N Engl J Med.* 1998;339:292-299.

Schnitzer T, Bone HG, Crepaldi G, et al. Therapeutic equivalence of alendronate 70 mg once-weekly and alendronate 10 mg daily in the treatment of osteoporosis. Alendronate Once-Weekly Study Group. *Aging.* 2000;12:1-12.

Risedronate
Borah B, Dufresne TE, Chmielewski PA, Gross GJ, Prenger MC, Phipps RJ. Risedronate preserves trabecular architecture and increases bone strength in vertebra of ovariectomized minipigs as measured by three-dimensional microcomputed tomography. *J Bone Miner Res.* 2002;17:1139-1147.

Brown JP, Kendler DL, McClung MR, et al. The efficacy and tolerability of risedronate once a week for the treatment of postmenopausal osteoporosis. *Calcif Tissue Int.* 2002;71:103-111.

Crandall C. Risedronate: a clinical review. *Arch Intern Med.* 2001;161:353-360.

Fogelman I, Ribot C, Smith R, Ethgen D, Sod E, Reginster JY. Risedronate reverses bone loss in postmenopausal women with low bone mass: results from a multinational, double-blind, placebo-controlled trial. BMD-MN Study Group. *J Clin Endocrinol Metab.* 2000;85:1895-1900.

Harris ST, Eriksen EF, Davidson M, et al. Effect of combined risedronate and hormone replacement therapies on bone mineral density in postmenopausal women. *J Clin Endocrinol Metab.* 2001;86:1890-1897.

Harris ST, Watts NB, Genant HK, et al. Effects of risedronate treatment on vertebral and nonvertebral fractures in women with postmenopausal osteoporosis: a randomized controlled trial. Vertebral Efficacy With Risedronate Therapy (VERT) Study Group. *JAMA.* 1999;282:1344-1352.

McClung MR, Geusens P, Miller PD, et al. Effect of risedronate on the risk of hip fracture in elderly women. Hip Intervention Program Study Group. *N Engl J Med.* 2001;344:333-340.

Reginster JY, Minne HW, Sorensen OH, et al. Randomized trial of the effects of risedronate on vertebral fractures in women with established postmenopausal osteoporosis. Vertebral Efficacy With Risedronate Therapy (VERT) Study Group. *Osteoporos Int.* 2000;11:83-91.

Reid DM, Hughes RA, Laan RF, et al. Efficacy and safety of daily risedronate in the treatment of corticosteroid-induced osteoporosis in men and women: a randomized trial. European Corticosteroid-induced Osteoporosis Treatment Study. *J Bone Miner Res.* 2000;15:1006-1013.

Wallach S, Cohen S, Reid DM, et al. Effects of risedronate treatment on bone density and vertebral fracture in patients on corticosteroid therapy. *Calcif Tissue Int.* 2000;67:277-285.

Watts NB. Risedronate for the prevention and treatment of postmenopausal osteoporosis: results from recent clinical trials. *Osteoporos Int.* 2001;12(suppl 3):S17-S22.

Other Bisphosphonates

Arjmandi BH, Alekel L, Hollis BW, et al. Dietary soybean protein prevents bone loss in an ovariectomized rat model of osteoporosis. *J Nutr.* 1996;126:161-167.

Diez-Perez A. Bisphosphonates. *Maturitas*. 2002;43(suppl 1):S19-S26.

Erdtsieck RJ, Pols HA, Valk NK, et al. Treatment of postmenopausal osteoporosis with a combination of growth hormone and pamidronate: a placebo controlled trial. *Clin Endocrinol*. 1995; 43:557-565.

Fleisch H. Can bisphosphonates be given to patients with fractures? *J Bone Miner Res*. 2001;16:437-440.

Giannini S, D'Angelo A, Malvasi L, et al. Effects of one-year cyclical treatment with clodronate on postmenopausal bone loss. *Bone*. 1993;14:137-141.

Harris ST, Watts NB, Jackson RD, et al. Four-year study of intermittent cyclic etidronate treatment of postmenopausal osteoporosis: three years of blinded therapy followed by one year of open therapy. *Am J Med*. 1993;95:557-567.

Kanis JA, McCloskey EV, Sirtori P, et al. Rationale for the use of clodronate in osteoporosis. *Osteoporos Int*. 1993;3(suppl 2):S23-S28.

Landman JO, Hamdy NA, Pauwels EK, Papapoulos SE. Skeletal metabolism in patients with osteoporosis after discontinuation of long-term treatment with oral pamidronate. *J Clin Endocrinol Metab*. 1995;80:3465-3468.

Landman JO, Schweitzer DH, Frölich M, Hamdy NA, Papapoulos SE. Recovery of serum calcium concentrations following acute hypocalcemia in patients with osteoporosis on long-term oral therapy with the bisphosphonate pamidronate. *J Clin Endocrinol Metab*. 1995;80:524-528.

Plosker GL, Goa KL. Clodronate. A review of its pharmacological properties and therapeutic efficacy in resorptive bone disease. *Drugs*. 1994;47:945-982.

Plotkin LI, Weinstein RS, Parfitt AM, Roberson PK, Manolagas SC, Bellido T. Prevention of osteocyte and osteoblast apoptosis by bisphosphonates and calcitonin. *J Clin Invest*. 1999;104:1363-1374.

12

Reid IR, Brown JP, Burckhardt P, et al. Intravenous zoledronic acid in postmenopausal women with low bone mineral density. *N Engl J Med*. 2002;346:653-661.

Reid IR, Wattie DJ, Evans MC, Gamble GD, Stapleton JP, Cornish J. Continuous therapy with pamidronate, a potent bisphosphonate, in postmenopausal osteoporosis. *J Clin Endocrinol Metab*. 1994;79:1595-1599.

Riis BJ, Ise J, von Stein T, Bagger Y, Christiansen C. Ibandronate: a comparison of oral daily dosing versus intermittent dosing in postmenopausal osteoporosis. *J Bone Miner Res*. 2001;16:1871-1878.

Storm T, Thamsborg G, Steiniche T, Genant HK, Sorensen OH. Effect of intermittent cyclical etidronate therapy on bone mass and fracture rate in women with postmenopausal osteoporosis. *N Engl J Med*. 1990;322:1265-1271.

Surrey ES, Fournet N, Voigt B, Judd HL. Effects of sodium etidronate in combination with low-dose norethindrone in patients administered a long-acting GnRH agonist: a preliminary report. *Obstet Gynecol*. 1993;81:581-586.

Thiebaud D, Burckhardt P, Kriegbaum H, et al. Three monthly intravenous injections of ibandronate in the treatment of postmenopausal osteoporosis. *Am J Med*. 1997;103:298-307.

Watts NB, Harris ST, Genant HK, et al. Intermittent cyclical etidronate treatment of postmenopausal osteoporosis. *N Engl J Med*. 1990;323: 73-79.

Selective Estrogen Receptor Modulators

Bjarnason NH, Bjarnason K, Haarbo J, Rosenquist C, Christiansen C. Tibolone: prevention of bone loss in late postmenopausal women. *J Clin Encocrinol Metab*. 1996;81:2419-2422.

Cranney A, Tugwell P, Zytaruk N, et al. Meta-analyses of therapies for postmenopausal osteoporosis. IV. Meta-analysis of raloxifene for the prevention and treatment of postmenopausal osteoporosis *Endocrine Reviews*. 2002;23:524-528.

Delmas PD, Bjarnason NH, Mitlak BH, et al. Effects of raloxifene on bone mineral density, serum cholesterol concentrations, and uterine endometrium in postmenopausal women. *N Engl J Med.* 1997;337:1641-1647.

Delmas PD, Ensrud KE, Adachi JD, et al. Efficacy of raloxifene on vertebral fracture risk reduction in postmenopausal women with osteoporosis: four-year results from a randomized clinical trial. *J Clin Endocrinol Metab.* 2002;87:3609-3617.

Kedar RP, Bourne TH, Powles TJ, et al. Effects of tamoxifen on uterus and ovaries of postmenopausal women in a randomised breast cancer prevention trial. *Lancet.* 1994;343:1318-1321.

Love RR, Mazess RB, Barden HS, et al. Effects of tamoxifen on bone mineral density in postmenopausal women with breast cancer. *N Engl J Med.* 1992;326:852-856.

Lufkin EG, Whitaker MD, Nickelsen T, et al. Treatment of established postmenopausal osteoporosis with raloxifene: a randomized trial. *J Bone Miner Res.* 1998;13:1747-1754.

Riggs BL, Melton LJ 3rd. Bone turnover matters: the raloxifene treatment paradox of dramatic decreases in vertebral fractures without commensurate increases in bone density. *J Bone Miner Res.* 2002;17:11-14.

Sarkar S, Mitlak BH, Wong M, Stock JL, Black DM, Harper KD. Relationships between bone mineral density and incident vertebral fracture risk with raloxifene therapy. *J Bone Miner Res.* 2002;17:1-10.

Calcitonin

Avioli LV. Calcitonin therapy in osteoporotic syndromes. *South Med J.* 1992;85(suppl 8):2S17-2S21.

Buclin T, Cosma Rochat M, Burckhardt P, Azria M, Attinger M. Bioavailability and biological efficacy of a new oral formulation of salmon calcitonin in healthy volunteers. *J Bone Miner Res.* 2002;17:1478-1485.

Dechant KL, Goa KL. Calcitriol. A review of its use in the treatment of postmenopausal osteoporosis and its potential in corticosteroid-induced osteoporosis. *Drugs Aging.* 1994;5:300-317.

Overgaard K, Hansen MA, Jensen SB, Christiansen C. Effect of salcatonin given intranasally on bone mass and fracture rates in established osteoporosis: a dose-response study. *Br Med J*. 1992;305:556-561.

Quesada JM, Mateo A, Jans I, Rodriguez M, Bouillon R. Calcitriol corrects deficient calcitonin secretion in the vitamin D-deficient elderly. *J Bone Miner Res*. 1994;9:53-57.

Reginster JY. Calcitonin for prevention and treatment of osteoporosis. *Am J Med*. 1993;95(suppl 5A):44S-47S.

Reginster JY, Denis D, Deroisy R, et al. Long-term (3 years) prevention of trabecular postmenopausal bone loss with low-dose intermittent nasal salmon calcitonin. *J Bone Miner Res*. 1994;9:69-73.

Reginster JY, Franchimont P. Side effects of synthetic salmon calcitonin given by intranasal spray compared with intramuscular injection. *Clin Exp Rheumatol*. 1985;3:155-157.

Sambrook P, Birmingham J, Kelly P, et al. Prevention of corticosteroid osteoporosis. A comparison of calcium, calcitriol, and calcitonin. *N Engl J Med*. 1993;328:1747-1752.

Silverman SL. Calcitonin. *Am J Med Sci*. 1997;313:13-16.

Siminoski K, Josse RG. Prevention and management of osteoporosis: consensus statements from the Scientific Advisory Board of the Osteoporosis Society of Canada. 9. Calcitonin in the treatment of osteoporosis. *Can Med Assoc J*. 1996;155:962-965.

Other Drugs

Brandi ML. New treatment strategies: ipriflavone, strontium, vitamin D metabolites and analogs. *Am J Med*. 1993;95(suppl 5A):69S-74S.

Hennessy S, Strom BL. Statins and fracture risk. *JAMA*. 2001;285:1888-1889.

Gallagher JC. The role of vitamin D in the pathogenesis and treatment of osteoporosis. *J Rheumatol Suppl*. 1996;45:15-18.

Jones G, Hogan DB, Yendt E, Hanley DA. Prevention and management of osteoporosis: consensus statements from the Scientific Advisory Board of the Osteoporosis Society of Canada. 8. Vitamin D metabolites and analogs in the treatment of osteoporosis. *Can Med Assoc J*. 1996;155:955-961.

Mandel FP, Davidson BJ, Erlik Y, Judd HL, Meldrum DR. Effects of progestins on bone metabolism in postmenopausal women. *J Reprod Med*. 1982;27:511-514.

Reginster JY. Miscellaneous and experimental agents. *Am J Med Sci*. 1997;313:33-40.

van Staa TP, Wegman S, de Vries F, Leufkens B, Cooper C. Use of statins and risk of fractures. *JAMA*. 2001;285:1850-1855.

General

Arjmandi BH, Alekel L, Hollis BW, et al. Dietary soybean protein prevents bone loss in an ovariectomized rat model of osteoporosis. *J Nutr*. 1996;126:161-167.

Cranney A, Guyatt, G, Griffith L, Wells G, Tugwell P, Rosen C. Meta-analyses of therapies for postmenopausal osteoporosis. IX: Summary of meta-analyses of therapies for postmenopausal osteoporosis. *Endocr Rev*. 2002;23:570-578.

Delmas PD. Treatment of postmenopausal osteoporosis. *Lancet*. 2002;359:2018-2026.

NIH Consensus Development Panel on Osteoporosis Prevention, Diagnosis, and Therapy. Osteoporosis prevention, diagnosis and therapy. *JAMA*. 2001;285:785-795.

Wimalawansa SJ. A four-year randomized controlled trial of hormone replacement and bisphosphonate, alone or in combination, in women with postmenopausal osteoporosis. *Am J Med*. 1998;104:219-226.

12

13   Drug Therapy Alternatives to Hormone Therapy: Bone Formation Stimulators

As noted previously, it is now clinically feasible to differentiate between high- and low-turnover osteoporosis by simply including the measurement of bone marker (Figure 13.1). There are at least three therapies that can be considered for low-turnover osteoporosis:

- Androgens and androgenic progestogens
- Sodium fluoride
- Intermittent parathyroid hormone (PTH).

Androgens

The biologic rationale for the anabolic effect of androgens on bone and muscle is discussed in Chapter 11. Studies based on this concept have documented why estrogen-androgen therapy as opposed to estrogen-alone therapy is preferable for the treatment of postmenopausal women with low-turnover osteoporosis—especially where other indications for the treatment of "nonbone" androgen deficiency (eg, decreased libido) is present.

Estrogen-androgen therapy is as effective an antiresorptive agent as estrogen-alone therapy but, in addition, it stimulates osteoblast function as measured by the enhanced synthesis and secretions of bone-specific alkaline phosphatase (Figure 13.2).

Estrogen-androgen therapy has a greater stimulating effect on the bone mineral density (BMD) of both the spine and the hip compared with estrogen-alone treatment (Figures 13.3 and 13.4).

FIGURE 13.1 — IDENTIFYING BONE REMODELING IMBALANCE

Bone Mineral Density (DEXA)		Bone Markers (Urinary collagen x-links*)
<	High turnover osteoporosis (> Osteoclast activity)	>
<	Low turnover osteoporosis (< Osteoblast activity)	<

Abbreviation: DEXA, dual-energy x-ray absorptiometry.

Both high- and low-turnover osteoporosis may present with equivalent reduction in bone mineral density. Measurement of urinary collagen excretion will differentiate between the two types of osteoporosis. High-turnover osteoporosis is treated with antiresorptives; low-turnover osteoporosis is treated with bone-stimulating drugs.

* Osteomark (NTx); Pyrilinks-D (deoxypyridinoline).

The minimal effective dose of androgen (testosterone) has not been established. From the only study available, it would appear that a dose of 2.5 mg methyltestosterone (or its equivalent) is optimum. There is, however, considerable interindividual variation, which may be partly due to the amount of endogenous androgen synthesis, the individual's ability to aromatize this androgen to estrogen, and the bone cell's affinity for androgens.

Methyltestosterone is not aromatized to estrogen. The positive influence of this drug on BMD may be due to a direct pharmacologic effect and/or the lowering of sex hormone–binding globulin (SHBG). This will result in the release of more bioavailable endogenous estradiol and testosterone.

Androgens are not approved by the Food and Drug Administration (FDA) for the prevention or treatment of osteoporosis.

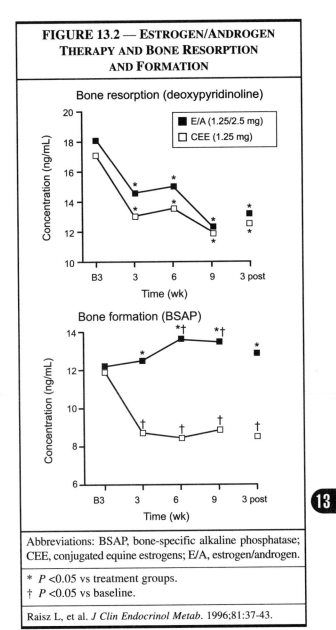

FIGURE 13.2 — ESTROGEN/ANDROGEN THERAPY AND BONE RESORPTION AND FORMATION

Abbreviations: BSAP, bone-specific alkaline phosphatase; CEE, conjugated equine estrogens; E/A, estrogen/androgen.

* $P <0.05$ vs treatment groups.
† $P <0.05$ vs baseline.

Raisz L, et al. *J Clin Endocrinol Metab*. 1996;81:37-43.

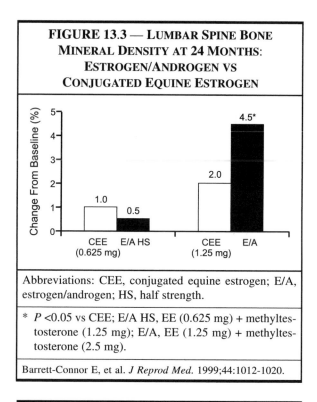

FIGURE 13.3 — LUMBAR SPINE BONE MINERAL DENSITY AT 24 MONTHS: ESTROGEN/ANDROGEN VS CONJUGATED EQUINE ESTROGEN

Abbreviations: CEE, conjugated equine estrogen; E/A, estrogen/androgen; HS, half strength.

* $P <0.05$ vs CEE; E/A HS, EE (0.625 mg) + methyltestosterone (1.25 mg); E/A, EE (1.25 mg) + methyltestosterone (2.5 mg).

Barrett-Connor E, et al. *J Reprod Med.* 1999;44:1012-1020.

Sodium Fluoride

Sodium fluoride is a drug with known bone-formation–stimulating properties but is not commonly used in clinical practice. This is due in large measure to the following three points that have characterized clinical trials:

- Excess dosage
- Prolonged duration of use
- Not combined with an appropriate antiresorptive drug (eg, estrogen therapy [ET]).

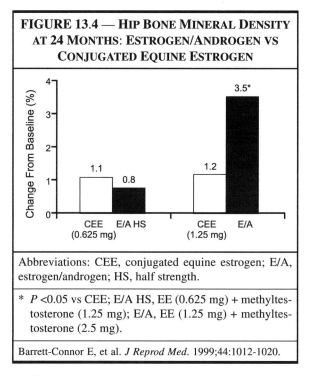

FIGURE 13.4 — HIP BONE MINERAL DENSITY AT 24 MONTHS: ESTROGEN/ANDROGEN VS CONJUGATED EQUINE ESTROGEN

Abbreviations: CEE, conjugated equine estrogen; E/A, estrogen/androgen; HS, half strength.

* $P <0.05$ vs CEE; E/A HS, EE (0.625 mg) + methyltestosterone (1.25 mg); E/A, EE (1.25 mg) + methyltestosterone (2.5 mg).

Barrett-Connor E, et al. *J Reprod Med*. 1999;44:1012-1020.

■ **Pharmacology**

Sodium fluoride is readily absorbed through the gastrointestinal wall by simple diffusion. Bioavailability is reduced by calcium and antacids; absorption is decreased by 20% to 50% if taken with supplemental calcium. Sodium fluoride is taken up more avidly at sites with higher metabolic activity; therefore, more is taken up by trabecular than by cortical bone.

Pharmacologic doses of sodium fluoride produce bone that substitutes fluorapatite and fluorhydroxyapatite crystals for hydroxyapatite, which is more resistant to osteoclast bone resorption. This is a dose-dependent phenomenon: "physiologic" doses promote hydroxyapatite crystals.

A therapeutic dose of sodium fluoride increases the number of osteoblasts. Depending on the dose, one may get a delay in mineralization of the matrix with resultant osteomalacia. Thus it is important to ensure adequate concomitant calcium and vitamin D supplementation. Lack of extra calcium can also lead to secondary hyperparathyroidism and cortical bone loss.

Effect of sodium fluoride on bone is dose-dependent:

- 200 mg/day sodium fluoride results in increased bone resorption and poorly mineralized new bone
- 60 mg/day to 90 mg/day sodium fluoride stimulates new bone formation with more normal mineralization if calcium and vitamin D are added to the regimen
- 20 mg/day to 40 mg/day sodium flouride, together with calcium, is the optimum regimen and should avoid defective mineralization of bone and secondary hyperparathyroidism. Avoid high doses of vitamin D, however, as this will accelerate cortical bone loss.

■ Effect of Sodium Fluoride on Bone Density and Strength

Vertebral bone mass can increase by about 10% per year. About 40% of patients show little or no response to sodium fluoride therapy. This may be due in part to noncompliance.

Fluoride-treated bone is more resistant to compressive forces but likely to fracture if exposed to torsional strain. Lower doses of sodium fluoride (50 mg/day with calcium and vitamin D) are associated with fewer new vertebral fractures.

■ Types of Sodium Fluoride

Appropriate formulations and doses of sodium fluoride suitable for adult use are not yet available. The following may be tried:

- Pediatric sodium fluoride tablets (2.2 mg per tablet): compound four to five tablets into one capsule to give a total dose of 8.8 mg or 11 mg sodium fluoride (elemental fluoride is half of this amount). Prescribe 3 or 4 times a day with meals, depending upon the dose required
- Sustained-release sodium fluoride (not FDA approved) plus calcium citrate supplement
- Sodium fluoride plus elemental calcium and a vitamin D_2 supplement (significantly lowered new vertebral fracture rate during second year of a 2-year French trial with no risk of nonvertebral fractures)
- Monofluorophosphate (MFP), now available in Europe (significantly increased vertebral bone mass in severely osteopenic women in a 2-year European trial; spinal microfractures were significantly more common in patients who received MFP than in placebo group).

■ Prescribing Sodium Fluoride

Based on the author's personal experience, the following clinical regimen is suggested:

- Limit the use of sodium fluoride to women with vertebral bone densities equivalent to ≤60% of young adult (<4 SD), and nonresponsive to hormone therapy alone.
- *Always* combine with:
  - Calcium, 1500 mg/day in the form of supplements (not to be taken together with sodium fluoride)
  - 400 to 800 IU of vitamin D
  - Estrogen: Premarin, 0.625 mg; Estrace, 1 mg; Vivelle, 0.1-mg patch biweekly, or equivalent.

13

(**Monitor blood estradiol levels to ensure a value between 40 and 60 pg/dL.**) Lower doses of ET may be applicable, depending upon pretreatment endogenous plasma estradiol (E_2) levels.

- Monitor the response to treatment by 6-monthly dual-energy x-ray absorptiometry (DEXA) tests of the spine and hip.
- Biochemical tests: bone-specific alkaline phosphatase; urine calcium-to-creatinine ratio; urinary collagen cross-links.
- If above parameters indicate increased cortical bone loss, monitor with plasma sodium fluoride levels. Values should be kept <0.2 to 0.25 mg/mL.
- Treatment (in responders) is only necessary for about 12 months to a maximum of 18 months. The bone-stimulating effect appears to persist for 2 years after stopping the sodium fluoride, provided that the patient is maintained on the above hormone, calcium, and vitamin D regimen.

■ Side Effects

The frequency of side effects varies with the dose of sodium fluoride, its formulation, and time of administration. Side effects include:

- Gastrointestinal:
  - Nausea
  - Vomiting
  - Pain
  - Diarrhea
  - Sometimes bleeding
- Osteoarticular pain
  - Dose dependent
  - Takes 4 to 8 weeks to resolve after stopping treatment

- May be associated with microfractures or stress fractures
- Occurs most frequently in patients with very low bone density.

Gastrointestinal side effects can be reduced by:
- Taking the drug with food
- Sustained-released sodium fluoride
- Sodium monofluorophosphate.

Sodium fluoride is not FDA approved for the prevention and treatment of osteoporosis.

Parathyroid Hormone

■ Biologic Basis for Anabolic Effect

Persistent and excessive secretion of PTH (as in both primary and secondary hyperparathyroidism) is associated with bone loss, especially in cortical bone.

Intermittent PTH has an anabolic effect and in animal studies increases the mechanical strength in trabecular and cortical bone by stimulation of new bone formation at the periosteal (outer) and endosteal (inner) bone surfaces.

The net result is:
- Thickening of the cortices of both types of bone
- Increasing the number and connectivity of the trabeculae.

Mechanisms of PTH action include the following:
- Induction of growth factors
- Increasing the cytokine RANKL and the osteoblastic modulation of osteoclast activity
- Reduction of osteoblast apoptosis
- Potentiation of osteoblast collagen synthesis.

13

PTH is an 84–amino acid peptide with its biologic activity located in amino acids 1 through 34. A recombinant form of human PTH (Forteo) has been developed of both the full peptide (recombinant human PTH [rhPTH] 1-84) and the active function (rhPTH 1-34).

■ Clinical Trials
PTH-Alone Therapy

rhPTH 1-34 was administered in two doses, PTH 20 μg and PTH 40 μg, by daily subcutaneous injection and the results were compared with a matched group of postmenopausal women treated with daily placebo injections. New vertebral fractures occurred in 14% of the women in the placebo group and in 5% and 4%, respectively, of the women receiving either 20 μg or 40 μg PTH (Figure 13.5). Lumbar spine BMD increased by 13.7% (PTH 40 μg), 9.7% (PTH 20 μg), and 1.1% (placebo).

PTH (both doses) reduced the risk of new nonvertebral fractures by about 35%. Markers of new bone formation increased significantly for 12 months and then returned to baseline (Figure 13.6).

PTH and Hormone Therapy

The rationale for PTH and hormone therapy (HT) is that the combination of drugs that have different mechanisms of action (antiresorptives and anabolics) should improve the quantity and quality of bone in an additive and possibly synergistic manner.

In women on maintenance HT (conjugated equine estrogen [CEE] 0.625 mg/day; transdermal E_2 50 μg; some with medroxyprogesterone acetate [MPA]) and PTH 25 μg, the lumber BMD increased by 13% compared with 2.7% in the control group, who continued with their HT-alone therapy. This increase in bone mass was associated with a significant reduction in vertebral fractures (Figure 13.7). This result has been confirmed by other studies using combination PTH and HT.

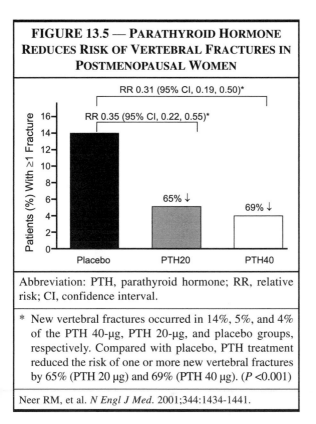

FIGURE 13.5 — PARATHYROID HORMONE REDUCES RISK OF VERTEBRAL FRACTURES IN POSTMENOPAUSAL WOMEN

RR 0.31 (95% CI, 0.19, 0.50)*

RR 0.35 (95% CI, 0.22, 0.55)*

Patients (%) With ≥1 Fracture

65% ↓

69% ↓

Placebo   PTH20   PTH40

Abbreviation: PTH, parathyroid hormone; RR, relative risk; CI, confidence interval.

* New vertebral fractures occurred in 14%, 5%, and 4% of the PTH 40-μg, PTH 20-μg, and placebo groups, respectively. Compared with placebo, PTH treatment reduced the risk of one or more new vertebral fractures by 65% (PTH 20 μg) and 69% (PTH 40 μg). (P <0.001)

Neer RM, et al. *N Engl J Med.* 2001;344:1434-1441.

PTH and Glucocorticoid-Induced Osteoporosis

PTH added to ET significantly increased the lumbar BMD in women with glucocorticoid-induced osteoporosis compared with ET-alone therapy. The increase in lumbar BMD persisted for 1 year after stopping the PTH therapy (Figure 13.8).

13

■ PTH and Trabecular Connectivity

Lattice distribution in trabecular bone determines bone strength without changing trabecular bone volume.

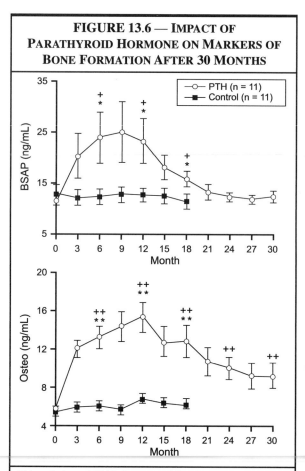

FIGURE 13.6 — IMPACT OF PARATHYROID HORMONE ON MARKERS OF BONE FORMATION AFTER 30 MONTHS

Abbreviations: BSAP, bone-specific alkaline phosphatase; OSTEO, osteocalcin; PTH, parathyroid hormone.

Markers of bone formation changed in a way that is very different from what is observed with the antiresorptive agents. BSAP and osteocalcin both rose remarkably during the first 12 months of therapy, but tended to return toward baseline.

Kurland ES, et al. *J Clin Endocrinol Metab.* 2000;85:3069-3076.

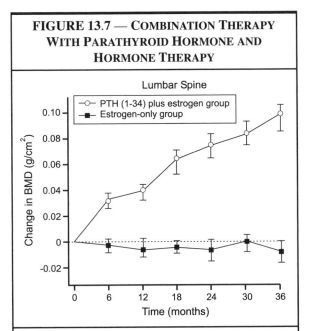

FIGURE 13.7 — COMBINATION THERAPY WITH PARATHYROID HORMONE AND HORMONE THERAPY

Abbreviations: BMD, bone mineral density; HT, hormone therapy; PTH, parathyroid hormone.

This 3-year, randomized, controlled trial evaluated the effects of PTH 400 IU (25 μg) in women taking maintenance HT and calcium 1500 mg/day. The cohort (n = 17) of postmenopausal women with T scores ≤-2.5 and stable BMD had been taking HT for >1 year. Bone mass increased at every site in the PTH-plus-HT–treated group, although the effect was most prominent in the lumbar spine (13%, P <0.02). In contrast, there was only a modest increase (2.7%, P <0.001) in total hip BMD. Increased bone mass was associated with a reduction in the rate of vertebral fractures (ie, a 15% reduction in vertebral height). Using the 20% reduction in vertebral height criteria, five fractures occurred in the HT-only group and one occurred in the PTH + HT group, P = 0.09.

Lindsay R, et al. *Lancet*. 1997;350:550-555.

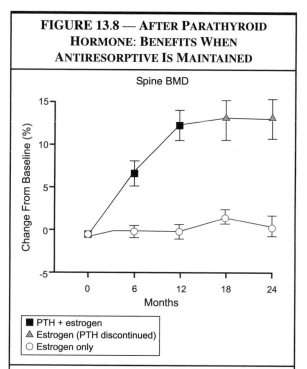

FIGURE 13.8 — AFTER PARATHYROID HORMONE: BENEFITS WHEN ANTIRESORPTIVE IS MAINTAINED

Spine BMD

- ■ PTH + estrogen
- ▲ Estrogen (PTH discontinued)
- ○ Estrogen only

Abbreviations: BMD, bone mineral density; DEXA, dual-energy x-ray absorptiometry; QCT, quantitative computed tomography; PTH, parathyroid hormone.

Significant improvement was noted in lumbar BMD as measured by QCT every year and by DEXA every 6 months (DEXA results shown in figure). The increases were significant at each time point. Biochemical markers increased more than 150% during the first 6 months, maintained their elevated levels throughout the treatment period, and returned to baseline values by 18 months.

Lane NE, et al. *J Bone Miner Res*. 2000;15:944-951.

> **Clinical Message**: BMD is not the only measure of bone mechanical competence.

Current therapies cannot reconnect disrupted trabecular plates. Histomorphometric study in iliac crest biopsies before and after treatment with 40 µg of rhPTH 1-34, revealed the following:

- Anabolic effect on cancellous bone volume
- Anabolic effect on cortical bone
- Increased connectivity between trabecular struts (Figure 13.9).

This study provides documentation of a structural basis for the reduction of osteoporotic fractures in women.

FIGURE 13.9 — PARATHYROID HORMONE INCREASES TRABECULAR CONNECTIVITY AND CORTICAL WALL THICKNESS

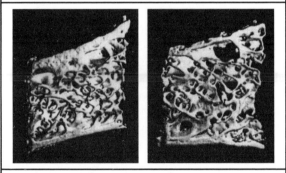

In these scanning electron micrographs of a 64-year-old woman, connectivity density and cortex thickness are shown to have increased after parathyroid hormone (PTH) therapy. Before PTH therapy *(left)* connectivity density was 2.9/mm³ and cortex thickness was 0.32 mm. Following PTH therapy *(right)* these measurements were shown to have improved to 4.6/mm³ and 0.42 mm, respectively.

Dempster DW, et al. *J Bone Miner Res*. 2001;16:1846-1853.

13

Clinical Interpretation

Advances in technology enable clinicians to identify patients at risk for osteoporosis (peripheral BMD), quantify the degree of bone loss in areas vulnerable to fracture (axial DEXA), differentiate between high- and low-turnover osteoporosis (bone markers), and based on this data, individualize the care of their patients by prescribing antiresorptives, anabolic agents, or a combination.

The development of digital topologic analysis as applied to magnetic resonance microimaging of the radius may soon allow for the assessment of an important additional link in the diagnostic armamentarium: the quantification of microarchitectural damage. This technology will provide a rationale for the use (and monitoring) of anabolic agents such as rhPTH 1-34. Thus present dogma that the disrupted microarchitecture of osteoporotic trabecular bone is irreversible will no longer be tenable.

Review of the data of available anabolic agents (androgens, sodium fluoride) based largely on clinical observation, experience, and short-term clinical trials, parallels that of the more appropriately designed and conducted PTH clinical trials. Two examples illustrate the point: androgens significantly increase levels of bone-specific alkaline phosphatase and the BMD-enhancing effect of sodium fluoride persists for at least 18 months to 2 years after stopping this treatment, provided the patient remains on HT and calcium plus vitamin D supplementation (personal observation).

Clinical Message: Long-term, randomized, clinical fracture trials involving androgens and/or sodium fluoride are unlikely to be carried out. Rather than discount these two forms of therapy for this

---

reason, clinicians should base their judgment on an understanding of the pathogenesis of osteoporosis, the pharmacology/pharmacokinetics of the drugs involved, and the needs of the patient. Often it is not the drugs per se that are ineffective (or unsafe) but the way in which they are prescribed. Clinicians should base their practice on a combination of clinical skill, personal experience, applied research data, judgment, and common sense.

SUGGESTED READING

Cosman F, Nieves J, Woelfert L, et al. Parathyroid hormone added to established hormone therapy: effects on vertebral fracture and maintenance of bone mass after parathyroid hormone withdrawal. *J Bone Miner Res*. 2001;16:925-931.

Delmas PD. Treatment of postmenopausal osteoporosis. *Lancet*. 2002;359:2018-2026.

Dempster DW, Cosman F, Kurland ES, et al. Effects of daily treatment with parathyroid hormone on bone microarchitecture and turnover in patients with osteoporosis: a paired biopsy study. *J Bone Miner Res*. 2001;16:1846-1853.

Dure-Smith BA, Farley SM, Linkhart SG, Farley JR, Baylink DJ. Calcium deficiency in fluoride-treated osteoporotic patients despite calcium supplementation. *J Clin Endocrinol Metab*. 1996;81:269-275.

Greenwald M, Brandli D, Spector S, Silverman S, Golde G. Corticosteroid-induced osteoporosis: effects of a treatment with slow-release sodium fluoride. *Osteoporos Int*. 1992;2:303-304.

Kanis JA. Treatment of symptomatic osteoporosis with fluoride. *Am J Med*. 1993;95(suppl 5A):53S-61S.

Langub MC, Monier-Faugere MC, Qi Q, Geng Z, Koszewski NJ, Malluche HH. Parathyroid hormone/parathyroid hormone-related peptide type 1 receptor in human bone. *J Bone Miner Res*. 2001;16:448-456.

13

Murray TM, Ste-Marie LG. Prevention and management of osteoporosis: consensus statements from the Scientific Advisory Board of the Osteoporosis Society of Canada. 7. Fluoride therapy for osteoporosis. *CMAJ*. 1996;155:949-954.

Neer RM, Arnaud CD, Zanchetta JR, et al. Effect of parathyroid hormone (1-34) on fractures and bone mineral density in postmenopausal women with osteoporosis. *N Engl J Med*. 2001;344: 1434-1441.

NIH Consensus Development Panel on Osteoporosis Prevention, Diagnosis, and Therapy. Osteoporosis prevention, diagnosis, and therapy. *JAMA*. 2001;285:785-795.

Pak CY, Sakhaee K, Adams-Huet B, Piziak V, Peterson RD, Poindexter JR. Treatment of postmenopausal osteoporosis with slow-release sodium fluoride. Final report of a randomized controlled trial. *Ann Intern Med*. 1995;123:401-408.

Pak CY, Sakhaee K, Rubin CD, Zerwekh JE. Sustained-release sodium fluoride in the management of established postmenopausal osteoporosis. *Am J Med Sci*. 1997;313:23-32.

Parfitt AM. Parathyroid hormone and periosteal bone expansion. *J Bone Miner Res*. 2002;17:1741-1743.

Riggs BL. Formation-stimulating regimens other than sodium fluoride. *Am J Med*. 1993;95(suppl 5A):62S-68S.

Riggs BL, Hodgson SF, O'Fallon WM, et al. Effect of fluoride treatment on the fracture rate in postmenopausal women with osteoporosis. *N Engl J Med*. 1990;322:802-809.

Riggs BL, O'Fallon WM, Lane A, et al. Clinical trial of fluoride therapy in postmenopausal osteoporotic women: extended observations and additional analysis. *J Bone Miner Res*. 1994;9:265-275.

Rubin MR, Cosman F, Lindsay R, Bilezikian JP. The anabolic effects of parathyroid hormone. *Osteoporos Int*. 2002;13:267-277.

Tashjian AH Jr, Chabner BA. Commentary on clinical safety of recombinant human parathyroid hormone 1-34 in the treatment of osteoporosis in men and postmenopausal women. *J Bone Miner Res*. 2002;17:1151-1161.

14

Established Osteoporosis: Nondrug Therapy

The prevalence of the morbidity and mortality of hip fracture is readily established. Women who fracture their hips are invariably hospitalized and thus fairly accurate statistics are available. For example, the estimated lifetime risk of hip fracture from age 50 years onward is 17% for white women in the United States compared with 6% in white men. Far more problematic, however, is the chronic pain—physical and psychological—suffered by countless thousands of women following vertebral fractures, few of which are treated in a hospital. Much can be done to prevent hip fracture and to improve the quality of life of women with spinal fractures through nondrug means. These include:

- Exercise (see Chapter 9)
- Physical therapy
- Hip protectors
- Vertebroplasty and kyphoplasty.

Physical Therapy

The principles involved and the methods of presentation and treatment have been succinctly summarized in *Walk Tall. An Exercise Program for the Prevention and Treatment of Osteoporosis* (Sara Meeks, Triad Publications, Gainesville, Florida, 1999).

Briefly stated, most back pain is due to three major lifetime factors:

- Poor posture
- Faulty body mechanics
- Weak back musculature.

14

287

The solution is to:
- Correct posture
- Develop good body mechanics
- Strengthen back muscles.

All of the above issues are exaggerated by the physical deformity and associated muscle pain that occurs with vertebral fractures.

Meek's program is based on six main goals:
- *Mental imagery:*
  - Dropping an imaginary plumb line from head to toe
  - Think tall
  - Maintain a level pelvis
  - Lengthen the midsection of the body
- *Site-specific exercises* to strengthen regional muscle groups
- *Balance*: evaluation and correction of problems with:
  - Vision
  - Hearing
  - Muscle strength
  - Posture
  - Relationship between the following:
    - Feet on the ground
    - Movement
    - Awareness of head position
- *Walking*: misalignment of the hip may be a significant contributor to low back pain
- *Scapular stabilization*: strengthening the scapular muscles is important for posture and relief of the frequently complained of "burning" back pain
- *Activities of daily living*, which include everyday activities and ways of ensuring that incorrect body mechanics do not aggravate the un-

derlying pathology. Guidance is given for how best to deal with:
- Standing
- Sitting
- Lifting and carrying
- Daily activities in the bedroom, bathroom, and kitchen
- Housework
- Yardwork
- Driving a car
- Pet care.

The importance of attention to activities of daily living cannot be overstated and will go a long way to aid the rehabilitation of patients with osteoporosis.

Hip Protectors

As illustrated in Figure 3.3, women who fracture their hip do so because they have lost both their sense of balance and protective reflex mechanism through loss of muscle strength and other factors. Instead of falling onto an outstretched arm (which usually results in a wrist fracture), they fall onto the greater trochanter of the hip. Other factors that contribute to the fracture include:

- Hip bone strength with bone mineral density (BMD) an important surrogate marker
- The mechanical stress and force of the fall
- The soft tissue energy absorption of the fall.

Hip protectors help to decrease the magnitude of the impact, and in one study, reduced the percent of fractures from falls by 85%. These data were generated from a study of 1801 men and women who were assigned to either wear a hip protector or not and were subsequently monitored for 18 months (Figure 14.1).

14

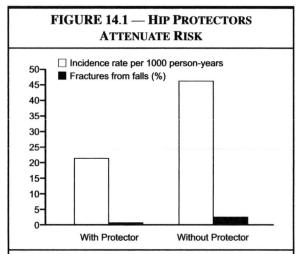

FIGURE 14.1 — HIP PROTECTORS ATTENUATE RISK

Legend:
- ☐ Incidence rate per 1000 person-years
- ■ Fractures from falls (%)

With Protector | Without Protector

Hip fractures are caused by a fall on the greater trochanter, and the components of the fracture include the fall, hip bone strength, energy absorption, and a protective reflex mechanism; often a wrist fracture may occur in trying to protect from a fall. Hip protectors are an extrinsic factor that can decrease the magnitude of the impact. They are indicated for specific patients, ie, those who fall easily, lean people, and those with previous fractures. Other patients also may be candidates for this type of treatment. Kannus et al showed that the number of hip fractures is halved when patients wear hip protectors (from 46.0 to 21.3 fractures per 1000 person-years). Similarly, the percent of fractures from falls is reduced by 85%, from 2.43 to 0.39 fractures per 100 falls. These data are from a study of 1801 ambulatory men and women who were assigned to either wear a hip protector or not and were followed for 18 months.

Kannus P, et al. *N Engl J Med*. 2000;343:1506-1513.

Vertebral Stabilization

Two procedures have been developed for the relief of pain associated with vertebral compression fractures. When successful, pain relief occurs within 24 to 48 hours and is quite dramatic. As further experience with these methods is gained, improved results with fewer complications can be anticipated.

Vertebroplasty is a minimally invasive technique and involves the placement of a special cement (polymethylmethacrylate) directly into the fractured vertebra, thus stabilizing the fracture (Figure 14.2).

Kyphoplasty involves the insertion of inflatable balloons into the fractured vertebrae, elevating the end plates, and injecting a bone cement into the decompressed area while removing the balloon. This technique involves general anesthesia and is most successful for the treatment of fractures in the T10 to L2 regions. It is aimed at both restoration of vertebral height and stabilization of the fracture. In some series, pain relief has been achieved in 90% of treated patients (Figure 14.3). Because the cement used in kyphoplasty is more viscous than that used in vertebroplasty, less complications occur.

REFERENCES

Belkoff SM, Mathis JM, Fenton DC, Scribner RM, Reiley ME, Talmadge K. An ex vivo biomechanical evaluation of an inflatable bone tamp used in the treatment of compression fracture. *Spine*. 2001;26:151-156.

Deramond H, Depriester C, Galibert P, Le Gars D. Percutaneous vertebroplasty with polymethylmethacrylate. Technique, indications, and results. *Radiol Clin North Am*. 1998;36:533-546.

Garfin SR, Yuan HA, Reiley MA. New technologies in spine: kyphoplasty and vertebroplasty for the treatment of painful osteoporotic compression fractures. *Spine*. 2001;26:1511-1515.

14

FIGURE 14.2 — VERTEBROPLASTY: VERTEBRAL COMPRESSION FRACTURE TREATMENT OPTIONS

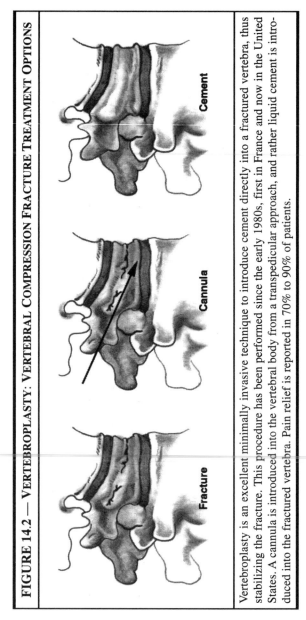

Fracture

Cannula

Cement

Vertebroplasty is an excellent minimally invasive technique to introduce cement directly into a fractured vertebra, thus stabilizing the fracture. This procedure has been performed since the early 1980s, first in France and now in the United States. A cannula is introduced into the vertebral body from a transpedicular approach, and rather liquid cement is introduced into the fractured vertebra. Pain relief is reported in 70% to 90% of patients.

FIGURE 14.3 — KYPHOPLASTY: NEW VERTEBRAL COMPRESSION FRACTURE TREATMENT OPTION

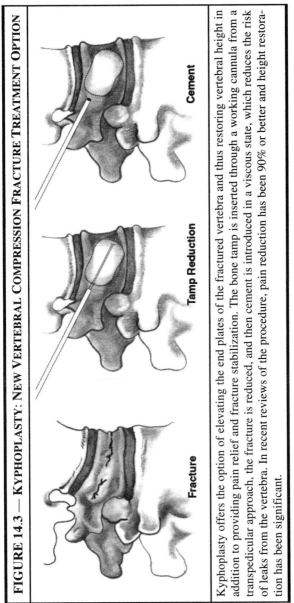

Fracture

Tamp Reduction

Cement

Kyphoplasty offers the option of elevating the end plates of the fractured vertebra and thus restoring vertebral height in addition to providing pain relief and fracture stabilization. The bone tamp is inserted through a working cannula from a transpedicular approach, the fracture is reduced, and then cement is introduced in a viscous state, which reduces the risk of leaks from the vertebra. In recent reviews of the procedure, pain reduction has been 90% or better and height restoration has been significant.

14

Jensen ME, Evans AJ, Mathis JM, Kallmes DF, Cloft HJ, Dion JE. Percutaneous polymethylmethacrylate vertebroplasty in the treatment of osteoporotic vertebral body compression fractures: technical aspects. *Am J Neuroradiol.* 1997;18:1897-1904.

Kannus P, Parkkari J, Niemi S, et al. Prevention of hip fracture in elderly people with use of a hip protector. *N Engl J Med.* 2000;343:1506-1513.

Lieberman IH, Dudeney S, Reinhardt MK, Bell G. Initial outcome and efficacy of "kyphoplasty" in the treatment of painful osteoporotic vertebral compression fractures. *Spine.* 2001;26:1631-1638.

Mathis JM, Petri M, Naff N. Percutaneous vertebroplasty treatment of steroid-induced osteoporotic compression fractures. *Arthritis Rheum.* 1998;41:171-175.

Meeks S. *Walk Tall! An Exercise Program for the Prevention and Treatment of Osteoporosis.* Gainesville, Fla: Triad Publishing Company; 1999.

Note: Page numbers in *italics* indicate figures;
page numbers followed by t refer to tables.

15

15

15

15

302

15

303

15

15

307

15

310

15

15

314

15

15

15